MW01631423

Extraesophageal Reflux

Extraesophageal Reflux

Edited by

Michael F. Vaezi, MD, PhD, MSc(Epi)

Professor of Medicine
Clinical Director, Division of Gastroenterology and Hepatology
Director, Clinical Research and Center for Swallowing and Esophageal Disorders
Vanderbilt University Medical Center
Nashville, Tennessee

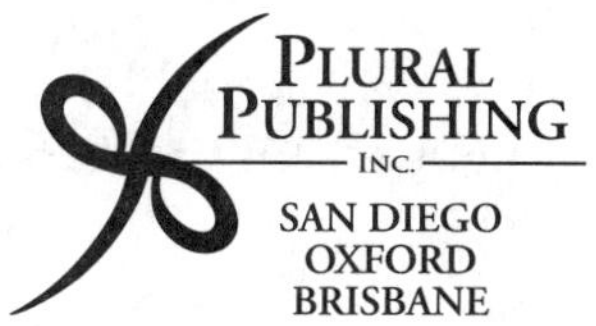

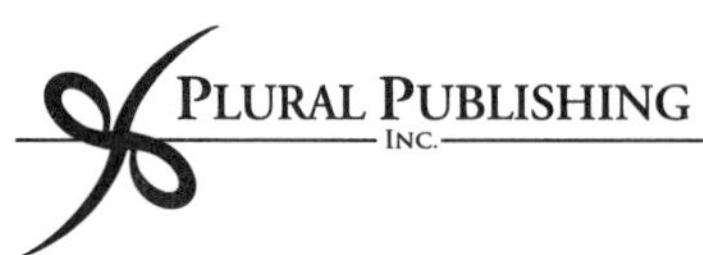

5521 Ruffin Road
San Diego, CA 92123

e-mail: info@pluralpublishing.com
Web site: http://www.pluralpublishing.com

49 Bath Street
Abingdon, Oxfordshire OX14 1EA
United Kingdom

Typeset in 10½/13 Garamond by Flanagan's Publishing Services, Inc.
Printed in the United States of America by Bang Printing

Library of Congress Cataloging-in-Publication Data

Extraesophageal reflux / [edited by] Michael Vaezi.
p. ; cm.
Includes bibliographical references and index.
ISBN-13: 978-1-59756-264-5 (alk. paper)
ISBN-10: 1-59756-264-5 (alk. paper)
1. Gastroesophageal reflux. I. Vaezi, Michael F.
[DNLM: 1. Gastroesophageal Reflux. WI 250 E96 2008]
RC815.7.E98 2008
616.3'24—dc22

2008035839

Contents

Preface *vii*
Contributors *ix*
Dedication *xiii*

1 **Epidemiology of Extraesophageal Reflux Disease** **1**
Millie D. Long and Nicholas J. Shaheen

2 **Pathophysiology of Extraesophageal Reflux Disease** **19**
Amit Agrawal, Neeraj Sharma, and Marcelo F. Vela

3 **Laryngitis: From the Gastroenterologist's Point of View** **37**
Michael F. Vaezi

4 **Laryngopharyngeal Reflux from the Otolaryngologist's Perspective** **49**
Paul M. Weinberger and Gregory N. Postma

5 **Laryngopharyngeal Reflux and Laryngeal Disorders: The Role of the Speech-Language Pathologist** **67**
Thomas Murry, Sabrina Cukier-Blaj, and Douglas M. Hicks

6 **Globus** **77**
Ted Mau, Dale C. Ekbom, and C. Gaelyn Garrett

7 **Asthma and GER** **93**
Susan M. Harding

8 **Gastroesophageal Reflux Disease and Cough: An Evidence-Based Approach to Diagnosis and Treatment** **107**
J. Matthew Bohning and Joel E. Richter

9 **Extraesophageal Reflux: The Sinonasal Passages and Middle Ear** 133
John W. Alldredge and Donald C. Lanza

10 **Dysphagia: Interactions with Gastroesophageal Reflux Disease** 151
David M. Shapiro and Ikuo Hirano

11 **Diagnostic Testing in Extraesophageal GERD** 165
John C. Fang

12 **Medical Therapy for Laryngopharyngeal Reflux** 185
Jonathan A. Schneider and Michael F. Vaezi

13 **Surgical Treatment of Extraesophageal Reflux** 193
D. Brandon Williams, William O. Richards, and Michael D. Holzman

Index 207

Preface

Gastroesophageal reflux disease (GERD), once a common and simple to treat disease entity, is no longer so simple to diagnose and treat. Patients' symptoms are no longer confined to heartburn and regurgitation. Many patients present with constellation of symptoms beyond the esophagus. *Extraesophageal Reflux* represents a group of syndromes in which patients present with symptoms not typical for GERD, such as: cough, asthma, laryngitis, globus, dysphagia, and even sinusitis and possibly otitis. Although the relationship between each atypical symptom and GERD varies, there are some common themes. In addition to the lack of the classic heartburn and regurgitation symptoms, esophagitis or Barrett's esophagus is usually not present. Additionally, response to antireflux therapy in this group of patients is often less predictable. The current practice of empiric therapy with proton-pump inhibitor therapy has unmasked a large group of these patients who do not show symptomatic response. The clinical dilemma in this group of patients is identifying which patient has GERD as the cause of the extraesophageal symptom in which patient GERD may be an innocent bystander or not at all present.

This unique book has compiled commentaries by experts in each of the fields of gastroenterology, allergy, otolaryngology, surgery, and pulmonary in order to best understand the current clinical challenges in this field and to help all subspecialties that interact with this group of patients. The state of the art scope of extraesophageal reflux is highlighted: epidemiology (Chapter 1), pathophysiology (Chapter 2), laryngitis from GI (Chapter 3), ENT (Chapter 4) and speech pathologist (Chapter 5) perspectives, globus (Chapter 6), asthma (Chapter 7), cough (Chapter 8), diagnosis and treatment (Chapter 8), sinusitis and middle ear (Chapter 9), dysphagia (Chapter 10), diagnostic testing (Chapter 11), and medical (Chapter 12) and surgical (Chapter 13) therapies. This book aimed to put together the latest developments and opinions from leading experts about a topic that encompasses different fields of medicine. It outlines diagnostic and management strategies for each of the above symptoms so that we can all better care for this group of difficult to diagnose patients. Based on the efforts of these contributors we have compiled a book that provides better appreciation of our current knowledge about this increasingly recognized disorder.

Michael F. Vaezi

Contributors

Amit Agrawal
Division of Gastroenterology and Hepatology
Medical University of South Carolina
Charleston, South Carolina
Chapter 2

John W. Alldredge, MD
Sinus and Nasal Institute of Florida, P.A.
St. Anthony's Carillon Outpatient Center
St. Petersburg, Florida
Chapter 9

J. Matthew Bohning, MD
Division of Gastroenterology
Department of Medicine
Temple University School of Medicine
Philadelphia, Pennsylvania
Chapter 8

Sabrina Cukier-Blaj
SLP, Voice Specialist
Master in Applied Linguistics
Research Associate at the Voice and Swallowing Center
Columbia University/New York Presbyterian Hospital
New York, New York
Chapter 5

Dale C. Ekbom, MD
Department of Otolaryngology
Mayo Clinic
Rochester, Minnesota
Chapter 6

John C. Fang, MD
Associate Professor of Medicine
Director of Endoscopy
University of Utah Health Sciences Center
Salt Lake City, Utah
Chapter 11

C. Gaelyn Garrett, MD
Associate Professor and Medical Director
Vanderbilt Voice Center
Vanderbilt University Medical Center
Nashville, Tennessee
Chapter 6

Susan M. Harding, MD, FCCP, DABSM
Professor of Medicine
Medical Director, UAB Sleep-Wake Disorders Center
Division of Pulmonary, Allergy and Critical Care Medicine
University of Alabama at Birmingham
Birmingham, Alabama
Chapter 7

Douglas M. Hicks, PhD, CCC-SP
Director, The Voice Center
Head, Speech-Language Pathology
Cleveland Clinic Foundation
Cleveland, Ohio
Chapter 5

Ikuo Hirano, MD
Associate Professor of Medicine

Division of Gastroenterology
Northwestern University Feinberg School of Medicine
Chicago, Illinois
Chapter 10

Michael D. Holzman, MD, MPH
Lester & Sara Jayne Williams Chair in Academic Surgery
Associate Professor of Surgery
Vanderbilt Medical Canter
Nashville, Tennessee
Chapter 13

Donald C. Lanza, MD, FACS
Director
Sinus and Nasal Institute of Florida, P.A.
St. Anthony's Carillon Outpatient Center
St. Petersburg, Florida
Chapter 9

Millie D. Long, MD
University of North Carolina at Chapel Hill
Division of Gastroenterology and Hepatology
Chapel Hill, North Carolina
Chapter 1

Ted Mau, MD, PhD
Assistant Professor
Clinical Center for Voice Care
University of Texas Southwestern Medical Center
Dallas, Texas
Chapter 6

Thomas Murry, PhD
Professor of Speech Pathology in Otolaryngology
Columbia University
College of Physicians and Surgeons
New York, New York
Chapter 5

Gregory N. Postma, MD
Director, Center for Voice and Swallowing Disorders
Professor, Department of Otolaryngology/Head and Neck Surgery
Medical College of Georgia
Augusta, Georgia
Chapter 4

William O. Richards, MD
Ingram Professor of Surgical Sciences
Director of Laparoendoscopic Surgery
Medical Director of the Vanderbilt Center for Surgical Weight Loss
Vanderbilt University School of Medicine
Nashville, Tennessee
Chapter 13

Joel E. Richter, MD, FACP, MACG
Division of Gastroenterology
Department of Medicine
Temple University School of Medicine
Philadelphia, Pennsylvania
Chapter 8

Jonathan A. Schneider, MD
Division of Gastroenterology, Hepatology and Nutrition
Center for Swallowing and Esophageal Disorders
Vanderbilt University Medical Center
Nashville, Tennessee
Chapter 12

Nicholas J. Shaheen, MD, MPH
Associate Professor of Medicine and Epidemiology
Director, Center for Esophageal Diseases and Swallowing
University of North Carolina School of Medicine
Chapel Hill, North Carolina
Chapter 1

David M. Shapiro, MD
Fellow
Division of Gastroenterology and Hepatology
Northwestern Memorial Hospital
Chicago, Illinois
Chapter 10

Neeraj Sharma, MD
Fellow
Division of Gastroenterology and Hepatology
Medical University of South Carolina
Charleston, South Carolina
Chapter 2

Michael F. Vaezi, MD, PhD, MSc(Epi)
Professor of Medicine
Clinical Director, Division of Gastroenterology and Hepatology
Director, Clinical Research and Center for Swallowing and Esophageal Disorders
Vanderbilt University Medical Center
Nashville, Tennessee
Chapters 3 and 12

Marcelo F. Vela, MD, MSCR, FACG
Associate Professor of Medicine
Division of Gastroenterology and Hepatology
Medical University of South Carolina
Charleston, South Carolina
Chapter 2

Paul M. Weinberger, MD
Department of Otolaryngology/Head and Neck Surgery
Medical College of Georgia
Augusta, Georgia
Chapter 4

D. Brandon Williams, MD
Assistant Professor of Surgery
Vanderbilt University Medical Center
Nashville, Tennessee
Chapter 13

To Holly, Lauren, and Blake whose love drives what I do daily

1

Epidemiology of Extraesophageal Reflux Disease

Millie D. Long and Nicholas J. Shaheen

INTRODUCTION

Gastroesophageal reflux disease (GERD) is a common disorder in the United States. In fact, approximately 40% of the population experiences heartburn on a monthly basis.[1,2] The true prevalence of the disease is likely even greater, as many patients with GERD do not have the "typical" symptoms of heartburn and acid reflux. Many patients also experience extraesophageal manifestations as well. Extraesophageal reflux disease (EERD) encompasses scores of potential otolaryngolic, pulmonary, cardiac and dental manifestations (Table 1-1).[3] Often the diagnosis can be challenging, as the patient may or may not have associated heartburn. Because of this, acid suppression is often used as both a means of diagnosis and of treatment.

There is a central contradiction in the literature regarding the causation by GERD of symptoms beyond the esophagus. Studies consistently demonstrate a strong epidemiologic association between extraesophageal manifestations and GERD. This may be related to the fact that common diseases often traffic together. However, the response to empiric treatment of putative EERD symptoms with acid suppressant agents or surgery has been inconsistent or nonexistent in controlled trials. This chapter briefly reviews the epidemiologic studies demonstrating the association between GERD and putative symptoms of EERD. Additionally, we discuss the literature documenting the response of these symptoms to acid suppressive therapy. Finally, we consider some possible explanations for this apparent contradiction. To organize this discussion, we rely on a widely accepted paradigm for assessing causality in epidemiologic studies, the Austin Bradford-Hill criteria, which are described below. Because there are a multitude of potential extraesophageal manifestations of GERD, and in order to organize the chapter in a logical fashion, we concentrate on

Table 1–1. Proposed Extraesophageal Manifestations of GERD

Pulmonary	Otolaryngolic	Cardiac	Dental
Asthma	Hoarseness	Chest pain	Halitosis
Bronchitis	Globus sensation	Arrythmias	Oral ulcers
Bronchiesctasis	Excessive throat clearing		Dental enamel erosion
Chronic cough	Dysphagia		Burning sensation
Idiopathic pulmonary fibrosis	Sinusitis		
Recurrent pnemonia	Sore throat		
	Laryngeal cancer		
	Pharyngeal cancer		

five extremely common potential manifestations of GERD: laryngitis, asthma, chronic cough, noncardiac chest pain, and dental manifestations of GERD.

Causality in Epidemiology

There is no single definition for causation in the epidemiologic literature.[4] The Bradford-Hill criteria[5] represent one set of criteria for determining causality that has been traditionally used in the field of epidemiology (Table 1-2). There are nine components to these criteria. The first of these components is strength. An observed association between a putative causative agent and a disease is more likely to be causal the larger magnitude the magnitude of the association. For instance, the relative risk for small cell cancer of the lung in tobacco smokers compared to nonsmokers is so large that the likelihood that such association occurred by chance is small. The second component is consistency. If an effect is stable from study to study, this supports a causal association. Next, specificity, or the ability of an exposure to repeatedly cause a single outcome supports causality.

The most important, and only required component of these criteria, is temporality. The cause must precede the effect. A common error in epidemiologic studies is protopathic bias, when the presumed "effect," or disease, actually precedes, and may compel the exposure. For instance, if pain from undiagnosed peptic ulcers led to individuals taking increased amounts of acetaminophen; epidemiologic studies might suggest a spurious association between acetaminophen and ulcers. The next criterion is a dose-response effect—more exposure to the putative causative agent should lead to a higher chance of disease, or more severe disease. Conversely, measures to reverse the exposure should display a graded protective effect. Plausibility of the effect is another component; the effect should be consistent with biological knowledge. It may be irrational to suggest, for instance, that a compound consistently known to be chemoprotective against polyps promotes colorectal cancer. Causal effects should also be coherent. The effects should not

Table 1–2. Austin Bradford-Hill Criteria for Causality in Epidemiology

Criterion	Description	Explanation and Example
1	Strength	A higher relative risk or odds ratio is evidence for causality; relative risk of lung cancer in smokers compared to nonsmokers is large
2	Consistency	Repeated associations support causality; association between smoking and lung cancer is consistent throughout studies
3	Specificity	Ability of an single exposure to repeatedly yield one outcome; asbestosis exposure is a relatively specific carcinogen for mesothelioma
4	Temporality	Exposure must predate the outcome; smoking after the diagnosis of Crohn's disease does not support an association between smoking and Crohn's disease
5	Dose-response	Higher levels of exposure should be associated with higher rates or more significant disease; higher levels of radon exposure are associated with increased rates of lung cancer
6	Plausibility	The effect should be consistent with biological knowledge; there is a proposed biological mechanism for NSAID use preventing colorectal polyps
7	Coherency	The effect should not conflict with what is already known about the illness; smoking has been shown to worsen Crohn's disease and therefore a study demonstrating a protective effect of nicotine would not be coherent
8	Experimental findings	Laboratory findings, including animal models of exposure, should demonstrate the exposure leading to the outcome; animal models with elevated cholesterol have developed increased coronary plaques
9	Analogy	Other explanations by inference; if cigarette smoking is known to precipitate alveolar inflammation and lead to bronchitis, a similar explanation might support the eventual development of bronchiectasis in such patients, buttressing the claim of a causal relationship between smoking and the disease entity

conflict with what is already known about the illness. Also, experimental findings, such as laboratory or clinical findings, should be supportive of causality. For example, a validated animal model of a disease state might be negatively impacted by exposing it to the putative pathogen. Finally, analogy or other explanations can be used as supportive evidence for causality. For instance, if cigarette smoking is known to precipitate alveolar inflammation and lead to bronchitis, a similar explanation might support the eventual development of bronchiectasis in such patients, buttressing the claim of a causal relationship between smoking and the disease entity.

Below, we apply selected aspects of these criteria to the data on EERD. We examine the definitions and prevalence of EERD in published studies in order to determine whether the proposed cause, GERD, precedes the extraesophageal symptoms. Although pathophysiology is covered extensively in another chapter, we briefly evaluate the pathophysiology of components of EERD in order to examine the biological plausibility component of the Bradford-Hill criteria. Most importantly, we discuss the treatment of each component of EERD with proton-pump inhibitors. This will allow us to investigate the several aspects of the above criteria, including strength, stability, coherence, and dose-response effect of treatment of reflux on EERD symptoms.

OTOLARYNGOLIC MANIFESTATIONS

There are many otolaryngolic manifestations associated with GERD. Some of these include hoarseness, globus sensation, excessive throat clearing, dysphagia and sore throat (see Table 1-1). Many of these symptoms are similar and are usually grouped under the heading of "laryngitis" in the literature. For example, patients have been considered to have laryngitis with a variety of symptoms including throat clearing, cough, globus, sore throat, or hoarseness.[6] Other studies additionally have looked at excessive phlegm and pain with swallowing.[7] Often, studies have used a composite laryngitis symptom score containing all of these symptoms.[8] The definition of laryngitis therefore is relatively imprecise and in most studies the temporality of GERD prior to the constellation of laryngitis symptoms has not been consistently established. Also, there is not specificity of the effect, thereby not meeting the Bradford-Hill criteria.

Laryngitis

Prevalence

Due to this variety in the definition of laryngitis, it is hard to determine the exact prevalence of these symptoms in association with GERD. In fact, there is a broad range in the prevalence estimate of GERD in those with laryngitis.[9] Case-control studies have shown an association between esophagitis and laryngitis.[10] It has been estimated that 4 to 10% of patients presenting to an ENT physician will have symptoms related to GERD.[11] As with other extraesophageal manifestations of GERD, many patients with laryngitis do not present with the classic symptoms of GERD such as heartburn or regurgitation.

Biological Plausibility

The mechanism of the association between laryngitis and GERD is considered to be related to acid and pepsin directly causing laryngeal injury. An alternative mechanism that has also been proposed is the "reflex" mechanism where esophageal reflux stimulates a vagally medicated response of throat clearing and coughing, which eventually could then lead to laryngitis.[6,12] It has also been proposed that these mechanisms of action both play a role in certain patients.[6] These mechanisms are biologically plausible and therefore do offer support for this component of the Bradford-Hill criteria.

Treatment

The first trial of acid suppression with proton-pump inhibitors for treatment of laryngitis was performed by El-Serag and colleagues.[13] They randomized 22 subjects with chronic idiopathic laryngitis to either active treatment with proton-pump inhibitor or placebo. A total of 20 patients completed the trial, and 50% of those on active treatment achieved a complete symptomatic response, compared to 10% in the placebo group (p = 0.04).[13] Since this original study by El-Serag, further studies have had trouble demonstrating a substantial therapy benefit of proton-pump inhibitors in patients with laryngitis (Table 1–3). Vaezi et al[8] published the largest study of proton-pump inhibitors in the treatment of laryngitis to date. This study of 145 patients randomized to esomeprazole or placebo demonstrated no significant improvement in laryngitis symptoms in the active treatment group as compared to placebo. Qadeer et al[16] recently published a meta-analysis of the role of proton-pump inhibitors in treatment of laryngitis. This study pooled data from 8 separate trials dating back to 1999. The primary outcome of the meta-analysis was the proportion of patients with at least a 50% reduction in laryngeal symptoms. The authors of the meta-analysis often had to go back to the original trial data as symptom improvement often was not an endpoint of the

Table 1–3. Summary of Randomized Placebo Controlled Trials of Proton-Pump Inhibitors in Patients with GERD and Laryngitis

Authors	*N*	Length of Therapy	Dose*	Results
El Serag et al[10]	22	12 weeks	Lansoprazole 30 BID	50% (*n* = 6) with symptom improvement in treatment group vs 10% (*n* = 1) in placebo group
Noordzij et al[7]	30	8 weeks	Omeprazole 80	Improvement in hoarseness, no change in throat pain, globus, phlegm, dysphagia, or odynophagia
Eherer et al[14]	21	12 weeks	Pantoprazole 40 BID	No difference in any symptom
Steward et al[6]	42	8 weeks	Rabeprazole 20 BID	No difference in total reflux symptom scores, health status, or laryngeal appearance
Vaezi et al[8]	145	16 weeks	Esomeprazole 40 BID	No difference in laryngitis symptoms
Wo et al[15]	39	12 weeks	Pantoprazole 40	No difference in laryngitis symptoms

*Dosing is QD unless otherwise specified.

original trials. The authors did evaluate for heterogeneity and publication bias in their analysis. No significant heterogeneity or publication bias was found. The analysis concluded that proton-pump inhibitor therapy did not significantly improve laryngitis symptoms when compared to placebo (*RR* 1.28, *CI* 0.94–1.74).[16] Without evidence of overall improvement of laryngitis symptoms with acid suppression, it is difficult to argue for a causal mechanism of GERD. There is not evidence of a strong effect, consistency of effect, or a dose-response effect of acid suppression in laryngitis.

PULMONARY MANIFESTATIONS

There are many pulmonary manifestations that have been potentially attributed to GERD throughout the literature. These manifestations include asthma, chronic cough, recurrent pneumonia, bronchitis, bronchiectasis, and indiopathic pulmonary fibrosis (see Table 1–1). The first two of these symptoms, asthma and chronic cough, have been extensively studied in the epidemiologic literature and are reviewed here.

Asthma

Prevalence

Asthma is a common disease with increasing worldwide incidence over the last several decades. Approximately 5 to 10% of the population is affected by asthma.[17] Epidemiologic studies have demonstrated an association between GERD and asthma.[10] Causation is more difficult to prove, as both disorders are quite common. Because GERD itself is a highly prevalent condition, it will be present in virtually any chronic disease population (Fig 1–1). In evaluating those with GERD, case control studies have shown that patients with objective manifestations of GERD such as peptic stricture and esophagitis have a greater likelihood of asthma when compared to controls.[10] In evaluating asthmatics, Sontag et al demonstrated that more than 80% of adult asthmatics in their Veterans' Affairs population had concurrent gastroesophageal reflux.[18] However, this does not necessarily support the temporality component of Bradford-Hill's definition of causality, as GERD did not necessarily precede the asthma in this group of patients. A recent large study in Norway of over 58,000 individuals demonstrated that people with asthma had 1.6 times the odds of having reflux compared to those without asthma (*OR* 1.6, 95% *CI* 1.4–1.9).[19] Interestingly, the reported prevalence of GERD in asthmatics has varied anywhere from 30 to 90% in the literature.[20,21] There are also significant numbers of asthmatics without any traditional symptoms of reflux who have abnormalities

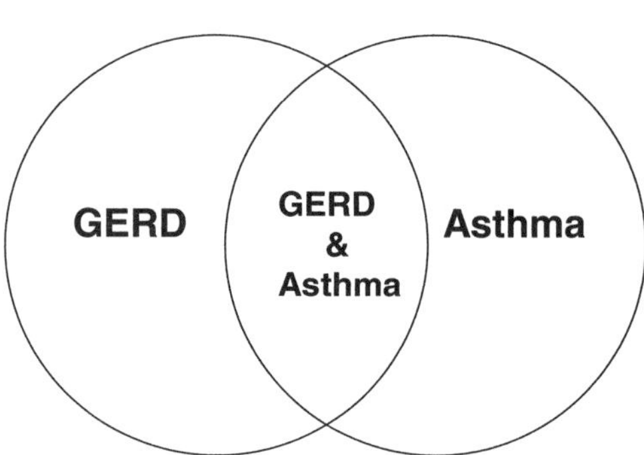

Fig 1–1. Prevalence of GERD and asthma may overlap, without inferring causality.

on pH-testing. Kiljander et al[22] evaluated asthmatics with 24-hour pH-monitoring in 2004. Approximately one-half of the total population had symptoms of GERD. Of those with symptoms, only one-half had objective evidence of GERD on pH-monitoring. In the converse situation, regardless of symptoms, one-third of the asthmatics had objective evidence of co-existent GERD. A significant proportion (1/4) of those with GERD had no symptoms of reflux.[22] It is unknown whether those with symptoms, but no objective evidence of GERD on pH-testing, were falsely labeled as negative by the pH-study. However, this study does demonstrate that symptoms of reflux and objective measurements on pH-testing in asthmatics do not necessarily correlate. There is no one single definition for GERD that is consistently associated with EERD symptoms. For this reason, the best means of establishing causality may be evaluating the effects of treatment with acid suppression on EERD symptoms, rather than examining pH.

Biological Plausibility

The primary biological mechanisms proposed in the pathogenesis of GERD-related asthma have included microaspiration of refluxed gastric and duodenal contents (including acid, pepsin, and bile acids) and a vagally induced esophagobronchial reflex.[3,12] The vagal reflex may be triggered by stimulation of vagal receptors in the distal third of the esophagus. These proposed mechanisms are biologically plausible.

It is also important to recognize, however, that there is good biological plausibility for asthma causing GERD as well. Subjects with asthma sometimes generate substantial negative intrathoracic pressures to inspire against bronchoconstricted airways. The generation of such negative pressures accentuates the pressure gradient that intragastric contents see, promoting reflux into the chest. By this mechanism, asthma may be a causal factor for GERD. The observed association may not be causal in the direction hypothesized, but rather in the opposite direction. The arrow may, in fact, point from asthma to GERD in a proportion of patients.

Treatment

There are 10 randomized controlled trials on the role of proton-pump inhibitors in asthma (Table 1-4).[23-32] Most of these studies are small and susceptible to Type II error. The larger trials have reached discordant outcomes. Even the definitions used for the diagnoses of asthma and GERD have differed in the studies. It is not clear that the GERD preceded the asthma, violating the criterion of temporality. The duration of treatment with proton-pump inhibitors has also varied, without evidence for an increased effect with higher dose or longer treatment with proton-pump inhibitors. Heterogeneous outcomes have also been used, including subjective measures such as symptom improvement or quality of life and objective measures such as rescue medication use or peak flow. Perhaps these differences in definitions and design have contributed to the lack of consensus in the literature and the lack of evidence for causation.

Only three of the aforementioned studies showed an improvement in peak flow with acid suppression.[23,26,27,32] One additional study demonstrated improvement in peak flow in the subset of patients with nocturnal symptoms.[32]

Table 1–4. Summary of Randomized Placebo Controlled Trials of Proton-Pump Inhibitors in Patients with GERD and Asthma

Authors	*N*	Length of Therapy	Dose*	Results
Ford et al (1994)[24]	10	4 weeks	Omeprazole 20	No change in symptoms or peak flow
Meier et al (1994)[25]	15	6 weeks	Omeprazole 40	No change in FEV1
Teichtahl et al (1996)[26]	20	4 weeks	Omeprazole 40	Improved peak flow, no change in symptoms, FEV1
Levin et al (1998)[27]	9	8 weeks	Omeprazole 20	Improved symptoms & peak flow, no change in FEV1
Boeree et al (1998)[28]	30	12 weeks	Omeprazole 80	Improved nighttime symptoms, no change in FEV1 or peak flow
Kiljander et al (1999)[29]	52	8 weeks	Omeprazole 40	Improved nighttime symptoms, no change in peak flow
Jiang et al (2003)[23]	30	6 weeks	Omeprazole 20	Improved peak flow and FEV1
Stordal et al (2005)[30]	38	12 weeks	Omeprazole 20	No change in symptoms, quality of life, rescue medication use or FEV1
Littner et al (2005)[31]	207	24 weeks	Lansoprazole 30 BID	Improved quality of life, no change in symptoms, peak flow or FEV1
Kiljander et al (2006)[32]	770	16 weeks	Esomeprazole 30 BID	Improved peak flow only in those with GERD and nocturnal symptoms

*Dosing is QD unless otherwise specified.

One study showed improvement in overall asthma symptoms.[27] One of the two studies that evaluated quality of life demonstrated an improvement.[31] These disappointing and conflicting results show that there may be a benefit of treatment in a subset of patients, but that improvement in asthmatic endpoints is not necessarily seen with treatment of GERD. These results do not support the Bradford-Hill criteria of strength of association, stability, dose-response or specificity of response.

Chronic Cough

Prevalence

GERD has been reported as a common cause of chronic cough regardless of age.[33] Chronic cough is defined as the persistence of cough for more than 3 to 8 weeks.[33] Among those with chronic cough, the likelihood that GERD is the inciting factor is estimated to be 11 to 43%.[34-38] The largest of these studies, the ProGERD study by Jasperson et al, found that approximately 33% of all patients presenting with heartburn had at least one extraesophageal manifestation such as chronic cough.[34] The range of prevalence in the literature depends on the patient population studied, whether pH monitoring was utilized to confirm the presence of GERD and whether other etiologies of cough were excluded.[39] There is therefore little evidence for the temporality, specificity, or consistency of the association.

Biological Plausibility

There are again two mechanisms for this association between GERD and chronic cough, the "reflux" and the "reflex" mechanisms. Esophageal reflux may be directly aspirated into the respiratory tract, thereby triggering a cough. There may also be a vagally mediated cough response that occurs in response to reflux.[12,39] These mechanisms again are biologically plausible.

Treatment

The association between chronic cough and GERD has been widely accepted by outpatient physicians,[40] yet there are few randomized placebo-controlled trials that have examined the effectiveness of proton-pump inhibitor therapy on GERD-related cough (Table 1-5). There are two small randomized placebo-controlled trials evaluating the effect of proton-pump inhibitors on chronic cough. Ours et al[41] randomized patients (n = 17) with a positive 24-hour esophageal pH test to placebo or proton-pump inhibitor for 12 weeks. After completing 12 weeks of blinded therapy, both groups were then treated for four weeks with an open-label increased dose of proton-pump inhibitor. In this study, only 1 of 8 patients receiving active drug during the blinded phase of the trial responded to treatment compared to no response from the placebo patients. However, 5 of 9 patients receiving active drug during the subsequent open label portion of the study responded to therapy. For this reason, the study was reported as a positive study, noting that 35% of patients responded favorably to treatment.[41] The limitations to this study include the small sample size and the fact that the patients who responded came from the open-label portion of the study. Artificially elevated response rates are common in any open label study. Kiljander[42] performed a

Table 1–5. Summary of Randomized Placebo Controlled Trials of Proton-Pump Inhibitors in Patients with GERD and Chronic Cough

Authors	*N*	Length of Therapy	Dose*	Results
Ours et al (1999)[41]	23	12 weeks	Omeprazole 40 BID	6/17 with positive pH test improved 0/6 with negative pH test improved
Kiljander et al (2000)[42]	29	8 weeks/ crossover	Omeprazole 40	12 patients on placebo then PPI improved 9 patients on PPI then placebo improved after PPI was stopped

*Dosing is QD unless otherwise specified.

randomized placebo-controlled trial of proton-pump inhibitor therapy for chronic cough in 29 patients with a positive 24-hour pH monitoring test. The study had a crossover design. The investigators found that cough improved significantly in those patients who received placebo first and active drug second. Those who received the proton-pump inhibitor first and placebo second, only showed improvement at the end of the placebo period.[42] Study limitations include small sample size, large attrition rate, and failure to analyze the final data using the original crossover design. Due to the small sample sizes and problems with methodologic rigor, it is hard to conclude that chronic cough in patients with reflux responds to acid suppression. This argues against a causative mechanism. There is no evidence for strength of the association or a dose-response effect.

CARDIAC MANIFESTATIONS AND NONCARDIAC CHEST PAIN

Two other often invoked manifestations of GERD are noncardiac chest pain (NCCP) and arrhythmias. The literature has focused upon noncardiac chest pain as this is a common disorder, affecting nearly one-quarter of the United States adult population.[43]

Noncardiac Chest Pain

Prevalence

Chest pain is a common complaint in outpatient, emergency room, and inpatient settings. After a complete cardiac workup is negative, patients with recurring retrosternal angina are labeled with the diagnosis of NCCP. When patients with NCCP are compared to patients with ischemic heart disease, they are usually younger and more anxious.[2,44] The etiology of NCCP is thought to be related to GERD approximately 60% of the time.[45] The disorder affects men and women equally, although women will often have greater contact with health care providers.[2] A population-based study in South America found the prevalence NCCP to be 23.5%, with an equal prevalence in men and women.[46] A similar estimate of the prevalence of NCCP was found in a Chinese cohort. In this study, GERD symptoms were frequently associated with NCCP (*OR* 2.3, 95% *CI* 1.7–3.1).[47] Dickman et al found the prevalence of esophageal erosions in patients with NCCP to be 24%.[48] Beeddassy et al[49] evaluated 104 patients with NCCP with pH-testing in order to determine the prevalence of GERD. They also correlated episodes of NCCP with abnormal pH. Approximately one-half of the patients with NCCP were found to have abnormal pH tests. However, only 21% of these patients experienced chest pain coinciding with abnormalities on pH-testing,[49] potentially arguing against a causative mechanism. There is also no evidence for temporality of this association.

Biological Plausibility

The underlying mechanism of NCCP in patients with GERD is not fully understood. It is thought to be related to a patient's reduced threshold for pain. Peripheral and/or central hypersensitivity may be associated with visceral hypersensitivity in these patients. Esophageal dysmotility is found in approximately

30% of patients with GERD and NCCP, although this is thought to play a limited role in their symptoms. Therefore, there is little evidence for a concrete biological association.

Treatment

After ruling out cardiac disease, treatment of patients with NCCP and GERD is with acid suppression therapy. Several small studies have evaluated the efficacy of proton-pump inhibitors in the treatment of noncardiac chest pain. Many of these small studies have demonstrated improvement in symptoms. One such study by Fass et al[50] randomized 37 patients referred by cardiology with NCCP to proton-pump inhibitor or placebo. All patients underwent 24-hour pH-monitoring and upper endoscopy in order to classify them as GERD positive or negative. This was a crossover study design where all patients received treatment for 7 days. A total of 23 (62%) were classified as GERD positive and 14 (38%) as GERD negative. A total of 18 patients with GERD (78%) had symptomatic response to the proton-pump inhibitor compared to 2 (14%) of GERD-negative patients.[50] Cremonini et al have demonstrated the likelihood of publication bias in the literature in a recent meta-analysis.[51] There are no published small studies with negative results. Therefore, the risk ratio may be an overestimate of the effect. These authors included 8 randomized controlled studies on proton-pump inhibitor therapy for NCCP. They found a pooled risk ratio for continued chest pain after PPI therapy to be 0.54 (95% *CI* 0.41-0.71). This demonstrates that a significant portion of NCCP does respond to acid suppression therapy. However, it is difficult to quantify symptom response in an objective matter. Table 1-6 lists the randomized controlled trials of proton-pump inhibitors in NCCP and the response

Table 1–6. Summary of Randomized Placebo Controlled Trials of Proton-Pump Inhibitors in Patients with GERD and Noncardiac Chest Pain

Authors	*N*	Length of Therapy	Dose*	Results
Pandak et al (2002)[52]	37	2 weeks/ crossover	Omeprazole 40 BID	53% with symptom improvement*
Fass et al (1998)[50]	37	1 week/ crossover	Omeprazole 40 AM Omeprazole 20 PM	78% with symptom improvement
Bautista et al (2004)[53]	40	1 week/ crossover	Lansoprazole 60 AM Lansoprazole 30 PM	78% with symptom improvement
Dickman et al (2005)[54]	20	1 week	Rabeprzole 20 BID	75% with symptom improvement
Achem et al (1997)[55]	36	8 weeks	Omeprazole 20 BID	81% with "overall" improvement
Xia et al (2003)[56]	68	4 weeks	Lansoprazole 30	53% with symptom improvement

*Defined as greater than 50% improvement in symptoms

rates in each.[50,52–56] The length of therapy in most of these trials differs, although it appears that symptom improvement often occurred quickly as many of the trials only evaluated 1 week of therapy. Most of these studies used the outcome of >50% improvement in baseline symptoms which is quite subjective. For those NCCP patients without objective evidence of GERD, or those who are unresponsive to trial of a proton-pump inhibitor, the mainstay of therapy is pain modulators to improve the visceral hypersensitivity. Although there is evidence of some improvement with proton-pump inhibitors, there does not appear to be a dose-response effect, nor is the effect particularly strong. These findings therefore do not support a strong causal mechanism.

DENTAL MANIFESTATIONS

Several dental manifestations have been attributed to GERD, including halitosis, a burning sensation in the mouth, tooth erosion and oral ulcers (see Table 1–1). The focus of the epidemiologic literature has been on dental erosion. The literature on erosion consists of both observational and controlled studies.

Tooth Erosion

Prevalence

The prevalence of dental erosions in patients with GERD has been evaluated in multiple case-control and cross-sectional studies. These studies show an increased prevalence of dental erosion in patients with GERD. This percentage has ranged from approximately 20 to 60%.[57–61] When patients with dental erosions have been evaluated for GERD in these small observational or case-control studies, the percentage found to have GERD has ranged from approximately 10 to 80%.[62–64] Meurman et al[57] evaluated one of the largest observational series of reflux patients, n = 117, and found 24% to have dental erosions. Oginni et al[60] performed a case-control study on 125 patients with reflux and 100 controls in 2005. Approximately 16% of GERD patients compared to 5% of controls had evidence of dental erosion.[60] Other small observational case series have found similar associations. In evaluating patients with dental erosion, Munoz et al[61] in 2003 performed a case-control study of 181 GERD patients and 72 controls. A total of 47.5% of the patients with GERD were found to have dental erosions compared to 12.5% of controls. The number and severity of the dental erosions also differed between groups.[61] Although these studies demonstrate an association between dental erosions and GERD, this is not necessarily evidence of causality. Again, GERD is common as are dental erosions, and common diseases traffic together. The association is also neither consistent, nor is it particularly strong.

Biological Plausibility

The primary mechanism of the association between GERD and dental erosions is related to direct acid reflux causing injury to the dental enamel. This can occur as pH levels drop in the oropharynx due to the acidic reflux, thereby dissolving the inorganic material of the teeth.[65] Therefore, there is biological evidence supporting causation of erosions by acidic reflux.

Treatment

Unfortunately, the effects of acid reflux on dental enamel are permanent and much of the treatment focuses on preventive strategies. Acid suppression therapy cannot restore the dental enamel. Preventive strategies currently employed include acid suppression with proton-pump inhibitors or antacids and rinsing of the mouth with neutral pH mouthwashes. Treatment for dental sensitivity includes desensitizing toothpaste or anesthetic mouthwashes.[65] There are no controlled studies randomizing GERD patients to proton-pump inhibitors in order to evaluate incident dental erosions. Without treatment trials, there is no way to assess the strength of the response to treatment, the consistency or the dose-response effect. Therefore, overall, there is little support other than a plausible biological mechanism for causation of dental erosion by GERD.

WHY WE SEE WHAT WE SEE: POTENTIAL EXPLANATIONS FOR STRONG EPIDEMIOLOGIC EVIDENCE BUT WEAK TRIAL DATA

We have discussed the recurring theme that multiple studies have shown a strong association between various extraesophageal symptoms and GERD. However, controlled trials have not consistently demonstrated a dose-response resolution of symptoms with appropriate therapy. There may be several reasons why this apparent contradiction exists. First, we may be observing spurious associations that have occurred no more often than would be expected by chance. Since many of the studies of association lack valid control groups, and as common diseases often traffic together, the observations may be nothing more than bias. Additionally, subjects who seek medical care for a given symptom are more likely to gather other concurrent medical diagnoses during their encounter with the medical profession. This might be the sum total explanation for the literature as we find it.

It is also important to appreciate that the literature on EERD is spread over multiple disciplines, including otolaryngology, gastroenterology, general medicine, pulmonary medicine, and general surgery. This has led to a plethora of disease definitions for most disease states. When trying to assimilate the literature on EERD, it immediately becomes apparent that definitions are not consistent: one investigator's laryngitis is another's normal control. Such heterogeneity further complicates attempts to draw conclusions from the literature, and may contribute to an apparent, but not actual, association between the conditions.

Study design and methodologic rigor differ substantially between studies and specialties. In some cases, GERD may be defined by presence of classic symptoms alone, allowing for substantial misclassification bias. Several of the association studies do not use pH definitions to define acid exposures.

Finally, and importantly, the lack of response to appropriate therapy in these studies may reflect our poor understanding of the pathophysiology of EERD. The association may, in fact, be substantial. We presume that EERD should act like classic GERD. We therefore assume that reducing intragastric pH should result in resolution of symptoms. Perhaps such simplistic reasoning is flawed. For instance, if the primary mechanism by which GERD causes asthma is through a vagally mediated reflex arc, perhaps deacidification of reflux is inadequate to affect this reflex, and asthma persists on that basis. In such a paradigm, the association is real, but the "yardstick" by which we are determining our dose-response relationship is flawed, leading us to spuriously reject the association.

CONCLUSIONS

GERD is a common finding in patients with asthma, cough, laryngitis, noncardiac chest pain, and dental erosions. GERD is present in patients with asthma approximately 30 to 90% of the time.[20,21] Nearly 10 to 40% of patients with chronic cough are found to have GERD symptoms and/or abnormal findings on esophageal pH monitoring.[34-37] Laryngitis and GERD coexist often, with a broad level of association estimated in the literature.[9] Noncardiac chest pain is present in approximately 20% of the population, and is attributed to GERD approximately 60% of the time.[45] Dental erosions are found in approximately 20 to 60% of patients with GERD.[57,59,60,63] With such a strong epidemiologic association in the literature, we would expect to find a consistent response to acid suppression. There are many observational case series that demonstrate symptom improvement in patients with GERD and extraesophageal reflux disease. However, when only the randomized clinical trials are examined, there is no consistent evidence of improvement in objective measures for the majority of patients with the evaluated extraesophageal disorders.

Important findings in the literature in regard to extraesophageal reflux disease include information on dose and length of course of therapy. If symptom response to proton-pump inhibitors does occur in patients with extraesophageal symptoms, often the patient requires a long course of therapy. Double dosing of the proton-pump inhibitor is often also required. The response to therapy is often substantially less than that with the typical GERD symptom of heartburn. Yet, there is not even consistent evidence that higher doses are associated with increased improvement in EERD symptoms.

In order to improve the quality of data on extraesophageal reflux disease, larger trials need to be performed. Also, definitions need to be standardized. Extraesophageal reflux disease needs to be defined with consistent pH criteria, laryngoscopy, impedance catheter, or other modalities. Even definitions by these modalities are limited. We rely too heavily on pH data to diagnose GERD. Host susceptibility issues also need to be considered. Outcome measures need to be standardized as well. In weighing the evidence using the Bradford-Hill criteria for causation, there is some supporting evidence that the symptoms of EERD may be caused by GERD, but overwhelmingly the criteria are violated. Although these symptoms traffic together, it is not clear that laryngitis, asthma, chronic cough, noncardiac chest pain, or dental erosions are directly caused by GERD. There is much remaining to be learned about the epidemiology, pathophysiology, and treatment of EERD.

REFERENCES

1. *A Gallup Organization national survey: heartburn across America.* Princeton, NJ: The Gallup Organization Inc.
2. Locke GR 3rd, Talley NJ, Fett SL, Zinsmeister AR, Melton LJ 3rd. Prevalence and clinical spectrum of gastroesophageal reflux: a population-based study in Olmsted County, Minnesota. *Gastroenterology.* 1997;112:1448-1456.
3. Vaezi MF. Atypical manifestations of gastroesophageal reflux disease. *MedGenMed.* 2005;7:25.
4. Parascandola M, Weed DL. Causation in epidemiology. *J Epidemiol Community Health.* 2001;55:905-912.
5. Hill AB. The environment and disease: association or causation? *Proc R Soc Med.* 1965;58:295-300.
6. Steward DL, Wilson KM, Kelly DH, et al. Proton-pump inhibitor therapy for chronic laryngo-pharyngitis: a randomized placebo-control trial. *Otolaryngol Head Neck Surg.* 2004;131:342-350.
7. Noordzij JP, Khidr A, Evans BA, et al. Evaluation of omeprazole in the treatment of reflux laryngitis: a prospective, placebo-controlled, randomized, double-blind study. *Laryngoscope.* 2001;111:2147-2151.
8. Vaezi MF, Richter JE, Stasney CR, et al. Treatment of chronic posterior laryngitis with esomeprazole. *Laryngoscope.* 2006;116:254-260.
9. Koufman JA. The otolaryngologic manifestations of gastroesophageal reflux disease (GERD): a clinical investigation of 225 patients using ambulatory 24-hour pH monitoring and an experimental investigation of the role of acid and pepsin in the development of laryngeal injury. *Laryngoscope.* 1991;101:1-78.
10. El-Serag HB, Sonnenberg A. Comorbid occurrence of laryngeal or pulmonary disease with esophagitis in United States military veterans. *Gastroenterology.* 1997;113:755-760.
11. Wong RK, Hanson DG, Waring PJ, Shaw G. ENT manifestations of gastroesophageal reflux. *Am J Gastroenterol.* 2000;-95:S15-S22.
12. Napierkowski J, Wong RK. Extraesophageal manifestations of GERD. *Am J Med Sci.* 2003;326:285-299.
13. El-Serag HB, Lee P, Buchner A, Inadomi JM, Gavin M, McCarthy DM. Lansoprazole treatment of patients with chronic idiopathic laryngitis: a placebo-controlled trial. *Am J Gastroenterol.* 2001;96:979-983.
14. Eherer AJ, Habermann W, Hammer HF, Kiesler K, Friedrich G, Krejs GJ. Effect of pantoprazole on the course of reflux-associated laryngitis: a placebo-controlled double-blind crossover study. *Scandinavian J Gastroenterol.* 2003;38(5):462-467.
15. Wo JM, Koopman J, Harrell SP, Parker K, Winstead W, Lentsch E. Double-blind, placebp-controlled trial with single-dose pantoprazole for laryngopharyngeal reflux. *Am J Gastroenterol.* 2006;101:1972-1978.
16. Qadeer MA, Phillips CO, Lopez AR, et al. Proton-pump inhibitor therapy for suspected GERD-related chronic laryngitis: a meta-analysis of randomized controlled trials. *Am J Gastroenterol.* 2006;101:2646-2654.
17. Woolcock AJ, Peat JK. Evidence for the increase in asthma worldwide. *Ciba Found Symp.* 1997;206:122-134; discussion 134-139,157-159.
18. Sontag SJ, O'Connell S, Khandelwal S, et al. Most asthmatics have gastroesophageal reflux with or without bronchodilator therapy. *Gastroenterology.* 1990;99:613-620.
19. Nordenstedt H, Nilsson M, Johansson S, et al. The relation between gastroesophageal reflux and respiratory symptoms in a population-based study: the Nord-Trondelag health survey. *Chest.* 2006;129:1051-1056.

20. Vincent D, Cohen-Jonathan AM, Leport J, et al. Gastro-oesophageal reflux prevalence and relationship with bronchial reactivity in asthma. *Eur Respir J.* 1997; 10:2255-2259.
21. Harding SM, Guzzo MR, Richter JE. 24-h esophageal pH testing in asthmatics: respiratory symptom correlation with esophageal acid events. *Chest.* 1999;115: 654-659.
22. Kiljander TO, Laitinen JO. The prevalence of gastroesophageal reflux disease in adult asthmatics. *Chest.* 2004;126:1490-1494.
23. Jiang SP, Liang RY, Zeng ZY, Liu QL, Liang YK, Li JG. Effects of antireflux treatment on bronchial hyper-responsiveness and lung function in asthmatic patients with gastroesophageal reflux disease. *World J Gastroenterol.* 2003;9:1123-1125.
24. Ford GA, Oliver PS, Prior JS, Butland RJ, Wilkinson SP. Omeprazole in the treatment of asthmatics with nocturnal symptoms and gastro-oesophageal reflux: a placebo-controlled cross-over study. *Postgrad Med J.* 1994;70:350-354.
25. Meier JH, McNally PR, Punja M, et al. Does omeprazole (Prilosec) improve respiratory function in asthmatics with gastroesophageal reflux? A double-blind, placebo-controlled crossover study. *Dig Dis Sci.* 1994;39:2127-2133.
26. Teichtahl H, Kronborg IJ, Yeomans ND, Robinson P. Adult asthma and gastro-oesophageal reflux: the effects of omeprazole therapy on asthma. *Aust N Z J Med.* 1996;26:671-676.
27. Levin TR, Sperling RM, McQuaid KR. Omeprazole improves peak expiratory flow rate and quality of life in asthmatics with gastroesophageal reflux. *Am J Gastroenterol.* 1998;93:1060-1063.
28. Boeree MJ, Peters FT, Postma DS, Kleibeuker JH. No effects of high-dose omeprazole in patients with severe airway hyperresponsiveness and (a)symptomatic gastro-oesophageal reflux. *Eur Respir J.* 1998;11:1070-1074.
29. Kiljander TO, Salomaa ER, Hietanen EK, Terho EO. Gastroesophageal reflux in asthmatics: a double-blind, placebo-controlled crossover study with omeprazole. *Chest.* 1999;116:1257-1264.
30. Stordal K, Johannesdottir GB, Bentsen BS, et al. Acid suppression does not change respiratory symptoms in children with asthma and gastro-oesophageal reflux disease. *Arch Dis Child.* 2005;90:956-960.
31. Littner MR, Leung FW, Ballard ED 2nd, Huang B, Samra NK. Effects of 24 weeks of lansoprazole therapy on asthma symptoms, exacerbations, quality of life, and pulmonary function in adult asthmatic patients with acid reflux symptoms. *Chest.* 2005;128:1128-1135.
32. Kiljander TO, Harding SM, Field SK, et al. Effects of esomeprazole 40 mg twice daily on asthma: a randomized placebo-controlled trial. *Am J Respir Crit Care Med.* 2006;173:1091-1097.
33. Irwin RS, Boulet LP, Cloutier MM, et al. Managing cough as a defense mechanism and as a symptom. A consensus panel report of the American College of Chest Physicians. *Chest.* 1998;114:133S-181S.
34. Jaspersen D, Kulig M, Labenz J, et al. Prevalence of extra-oesophageal manifestations in gastro-oesophageal reflux disease: an analysis based on the ProGERD Study. *Aliment Pharmacol Ther.* 2003; 17:1515-1520.
35. Pratter MR, Bartter T, Akers S, DuBois J. An algorithmic approach to chronic cough. *Ann Intern Med.* 1993;119: 977-983.
36. Smyrnios NA, Irwin RS, Curley FJ. Chronic cough with a history of excessive sputum production. The spectrum and frequency of causes, key components of the diagnostic evaluation, and outcome of specific therapy. *Chest.* 1995;108:991-997.
37. Smyrnios NA, Irwin RS, Curley FJ, French CL. From a prospective study of chronic cough: diagnostic and therapeutic aspects in older adults. *Arch Intern Med.* 1998; 158:1222-1228.
38. Poe RH, Kallay MC. Chronic cough and gastroesophageal reflux disease: experi-

ence with specific therapy for diagnosis and treatment. *Chest.* 2003;123:679-684.

39. Harding SM, Richter JE. The role of gastroesophageal reflux in chronic cough and asthma. *Chest.* 1997;111:1389-1402.
40. Slusarcick AL, McCaig LF. National Hospital Ambulatory Medical Care Survey: 1998 outpatient department summary. *Adv Data.* 2000:1-23.
41. Ours TM, Kavuru MS, Schilz RJ, Richter JE. A prospective evaluation of esophageal testing and a double-blind, randomized study of omeprazole in a diagnostic and therapeutic algorithm for chronic cough. *Am J Gastroenterol.* 1999;94:3131-3138.
42. Kiljander TO, Salomaa ER, Hietanen EK, Terho EO. Chronic cough and gastro-oesophageal reflux: a double-blind placebo-controlled study with omeprazole. *Eur Respir J.* 2000;16:633-638.
43. Fass R, Dickman R. Non-cardiac chest pain: an update. *Neurogastroenterol Motil.* 2006;18:408-417.
44. Tew R, Guthrie EA, Creed FH, Cotter L, Kisely S, Tomenson B. A long-term follow-up study of patients with ischaemic heart disease versus patients with nonspecific chest pain. *J Psychosom Res.* 1995;39:977-985.
45. Hewson EG, Sinclair JW, Dalton CB, Richter JE. Twenty-four-hour esophageal pH monitoring: the most useful test for evaluating noncardiac chest pain. *Am J Med.* 1991;90:576-583.
46. Chiocca JC, Olmos JA, Salis GB, Soifer LO, Higa R, Marcolongo M. Prevalence, clinical spectrum and atypical symptoms of gastro-oesophageal reflux in Argentina: a nationwide population-based study. *Aliment Pharmacol Ther.* 2005;22:331-342.
47. Wong WM, Lai KC, Lam KF, et al. Prevalence, clinical spectrum and health care utilization of gastro-oesophageal reflux disease in a Chinese population: a population-based study. *Aliment Pharmacol Ther.* 2003;18:595-604.
48. Dickman R, Mattek N, Holub J, Peters D, Fass R. Prevalence of upper gastrointestinal tract findings in patients with noncardiac chest pain versus those with gastroesophageal reflux disease (GERD)-related symptoms: results from a national endoscopic database. *Am J Gastroenterol.* 2007;102:1173-1179.
49. Beedassy A, Katz PO, Gruber A, Peghini PL, Castell DO. Prior sensitization of esophageal mucosa by acid reflux predisposes to reflux-induced chest pain. *J Clin Gastroenterol.* 2000;31:121-124.
50. Fass R, Fennerty MB, Ofman JJ, et al. The clinical and economic value of a short course of omeprazole in patients with noncardiac chest pain. *Gastroenterology.* 1998;115:42-49.
51. Cremonini F, Wise J, Moayyedi P, Talley NJ. Diagnostic and therapeutic use of proton-pump inhibitors in non-cardiac chest pain: a metaanalysis. *Am J Gastroenterol.* 2005;100:1226-1232.
52. Pandak WM, Arezo S, Everett S, et al. Short course of omeprazole: a better first diagnostic approach to noncardiac chest pain than endoscopy, manometry, or 24-hour esophageal pH monitoring. *J Clin Gastroenterol.* 2002;35:307-314.
53. Bautista J, Fullerton H, Briseno M, Cui H, Fass R. The effect of an empirical trial of high-dose lansoprazole on symptom response of patients with non-cardiac chest pain—a randomized, double-blind, placebo-controlled, crossover trial. *Aliment Pharmacol Ther.* 2004;19:1123-1130.
54. Dickman R, Emmons S, Cui H, et al. The effect of a therapeutic trial of high-dose rabeprazole on symptom response of patients with non-cardiac chest pain: a randomized, double-blind, placebo-controlled, crossover trial. *Aliment Pharmacol Ther.* 2005;22:547-555.
55. Achem SR, Kolts BE, MacMath T, et al. Effects of omeprazole versus placebo in treatment of noncardiac chest pain and gastroesophageal reflux. *Dig Dis Sci.* 1997;42:2138-2145.
56. Xia HH, Lai KC, Lam SK, et al. Symptomatic response to lansoprazole predicts

abnormal acid reflux in endoscopy-negative patients with non-cardiac chest pain. *Aliment Pharmacol Ther.* 2003; 17:369-377.

57. Meurman JH, Toskala J, Nuutinen P, Klemetti E. Oral and dental manifestations in gastroesophageal reflux disease. *Oral Surg Oral Med Oral Pathol.* 1994; 78:583-589.
58. Moazzez R, Bartlett D, Anggiansah A. Dental erosion, gastro-oesophageal reflux disease and saliva: how are they related? *J Dent.* 2004;32:489-494.
59. Jarvinen V, Meurman JH, Hyvarinen H, Rytomaa I, Murtomaa H. Dental erosion and upper gastrointestinal disorders. *Oral Surg Oral Med Oral Pathol.* 1988; 65:298-303.
60. Oginni AO, Agbakwuru EA, Ndububa DA. The prevalence of dental erosion in Nigerian patients with gastro-oesophageal reflux disease. *BMC Oral Health.* 2005;5:1.
61. Munoz JV, Herreros B, Sanchiz V, et al. Dental and periodontal lesions in patients with gastro-oesophageal reflux disease. *Dig Liver Dis.* 2003;35:461-467.
62. Schroeder PL, Filler SJ, Ramirez B, Lazarchik DA, Vaezi MF, Richter JE. Dental erosion and acid reflux disease. *Ann Intern Med.* 1995;122:809-815.
63. Bartlett DW, Evans DF, Smith BG. The relationship between gastro-oesophageal reflux disease and dental erosion. *J Oral Rehabil.* 1996;23:289-297.
64. Ali DA, Brown RS, Rodriguez LO, Moody EL, Nasr MF. Dental erosion caused by silent gastroesophageal reflux disease. *J Am Dent Assoc.* 2002;133:734-737; quiz 768-769.
65. Farrokhi F, Vaezi MF. Extraesophageal manifestations of gastroesophageal reflux. *Oral Dis.* 2007;13:349-359.

2

Pathophysiology of Extraesophageal Reflux Disease

Amit Agrawal, Neeraj Sharma, and Marcelo F. Vela

INTRODUCTION

Gastroesophageal reflux disease (GERD), defined as the presence of symptoms or mucosal damage that can be attributed to the reflux of stomach contents into the esophagus or supraesophageal structures, is a common clinical problem affecting all segments of the population. Nearly 20% of Americans experience heartburn or acid regurgitation weekly with an annual prevalence of up to 59%.[1] Over the last several years, GERD has been increasingly recognized as a potential cause of laryngeal and pulmonary disease. This chapter focuses on the pathophysiology of GERD in general and the mechanisms leading to GERD-related injury to the larynx and the lungs.

PATHOPHYSIOLOGY OF GERD

Reflux of gastric contents into the esophagus occurs as a result of the interplay among different factors in the upper gastrointestinal tract (Color Plate 1). Potentially harmful agents to the esophageal mucosa include gastric (acid and pepsin) or duodenal (conjugated and unconjugated bile acids and trypsin) secretions. The lower esophageal sphincter (LES), in concert with the crural diaphragm forms a barrier at the gastroesophageal junction in order to prevent movement of harmful gastroduodenal contents into the esophagus. This barrier may be breached as a result of transient lower esophageal relaxations (TLESRs), hypotensive LES, or other mechanisms associated with the presence of a hiatal hernia. Once esophageal mucosa is exposed to the damaging gastroduodenal agents luminal protection occurs through esophageal clearance (through peristalsis) as well as mechanisms of epithelial defense and repair, in order to prevent mucosal injury. When the barrier at the esophagogastric junction is breached frequently, such that the protective mechanisms in the esophagus are overwhelmed by the harmful gastroduodenal contents, the patient will develop symptoms. In addition, some but not all patients will develop visible signs of epithelial damage, either in the esophagus or in supraesophageal structures.

Gastroduodenal Factors

The most injurious gastric components are acid produced by the parietal cells and pepsin produced by the gastric chief cells. These gastric contents may be mixed with duodenal material containing bile acids and trypsin. Additional factors that contribute to the pathogenesis of GERD in the stomach are *H. pylori* which can have an impact on gastric acid secretion, and the degree of gastric emptying.

Acid and Pepsin

Substantial experimental and clinical evidence strongly supports the importance of acid and pepsin in GERD.[2] Animal experiments have shown that acid alone may cause injury to the esophageal mucosa only at very low pH values (pH 1–2). On the other hand, the combination of acid and even small concentrations of pepsin results in macroscopic as well as microscopic esophageal injury.[3] Acid results in cellular damage because a high concentration of hydrogen ions impairs cell volume regulation leading to edema and ultimately necrosis.[4] Pepsin, once activated in and acidic milieu (pH <4), can damage the esophagus by proteolysis (it is inactive at pH >4.0).[5] Early investigations[6] measuring distal esophageal acid exposure have shown good correlation between symptomatic heartburn and esophageal exposure to reflux material with pH <4. Additionally, a series of studies[7–11] have shown that patients with various grades of esophagitis, including Barrett's esophagus, have increased frequency and duration of esophageal exposure to refluxate with pH <4. Interestingly, while increased exposure to acid in the esophagus has been clearly demonstrated in subjects with GERD, production of acid in the stomach is not increased in these patients. This was demonstrated by Hirschowitz et al,[12] who found that basal and pentagastrin-stimulated secretion of gastric acid and pepsin was similar between GERD patients and healthy controls. Therefore, the abnormal esophageal acid exposure in GERD identified on ambulatory pH monitoring is most likely due to failure of the gastroesophageal barrier and poor esophageal clearance (discussed below). That said, there is a small number of patients, such as those with Zollinger-Ellison syndrome, in whom hypersecretion of acid leads to increased gastroesophageal reflux.[13]

Biliary and Pancreatic Secretions

Bile acids and pancreatic enzymes may migrate from the duodenum, across the pylorus and into the stomach, where they intermix with gastric secretions. The role of these duodenal contents in the development of esophageal mucosal injury is controversial and the subject of many in vitro animal studies.[14-18] These studies suggest that the esophageal mucosal damage is dependent on the conjugation state of the bile acids. Conjugated forms are injurious at an acidic pH, whereas unconjugated forms are harmful at alkaline pH ranges. The way in which bile produces mucosal injury is not well understood; proposed mechanisms include cell damage through solubilization of the mucosal lipid membranes and intramucosal damage after entry of bile salts into the cell. Trypsin, like pepsin, harms through proteolysis and is most injurious at a pH range between 5 and 8.[19] The clinical evidence for the possible damaging effects of duodenogastroesophageal reflux (DGER) on the esophageal mucosa remains controversial. However, recent studies by Vaezi and Richter[20] using the ambulatory bilirubin monitoring device (Bilitec) suggests that DGER parallels acid reflux in the clinical spectrum of GERD, being highest in patients with Barrett's esophagus. Furthermore, these investigators found that simultaneous esophageal exposure to both acid and DGER was the most prevalent reflux pattern occurring in 95% of patients with Barrett's esophagus and 79% of GERD patients. In fact, they found a strong correlation (R = 0.73) between acid and DGER in controls, reflux patients, and those with Barrett's esophagus. Thus, these studies support the earlier findings in animals that suggested a possible synergy between acid and bile acids in the development of esophagitis and Barrett's esophagus.

The role of DGER in producing esophageal mucosal injury, in the absence of acid reflux, was not clarified until recently. Studies by Marshall et al[21] using prolonged pH and bilirubin monitoring in 38 patients with GERD found that DGER in the absence of acid reflux was a rare event (7%) in patients without prior gastric surgery. Additionally, Sears and colleagues[22] studied 13 partial gastrectomy patients with reflux symptoms and found increased DGER by Bilitec monitoring in 77% of patients. Endoscopic esophagitis, however, was present only in those who had concomitant acid reflux. Subsequently, Vaezi et al[23] confirmed these observations and found that only 24% of upper gastrointestinal symptoms reported by partial gastrectomy patients were due to DGER in the absence of acid reflux. These studies show that DGER without excessive acid reflux can cause reflux symptoms but does not usually produce esophagitis.

Therefore, studies suggest that acid and pepsin are by far the main culprits behind mucosal injury. Duodenal contents contribute to mucosal damage in the presence of acid and pepsin, but in their absence may not be injurious. However, reflux of nonacidic gastroduodenal contents may be responsible for continued symptoms in some patients treated with acid suppressing medications. Using combined pH and bilirubin monitoring Koek et al[24] showed that in 15 symptomatic patients treated with proton-pump inhibitors, bile reflux elicited GERD symptoms. In a study using the recently developed technique of combined intraluminal impedance and pH, which allows measurement of both acid and nonacid reflux, Vela et al[25] reported that in a group of subjects with frequent heartburn studied in the postprandial period, omeprazole significantly decreased the number of acid reflux episodes; however, nonacid reflux continued to occur and was responsible for some symptoms. The importance of bile and nonacid reflux in symptomatic patients, particularly those with adequate acid suppression, awaits further study. Studies using multichannel intraluminal impedance which is capable of differentiating between liquid and gas, as well as acid and nonacid reflux, are likely to expand our knowledge in this area.

Gastric Emptying

Delayed gastric emptying may result in increased gastroesophageal reflux by triggering transient LES relaxations (TLESRs), which constitute one of the main mechanisms underlying reflux, as explained below. Although studies evaluating the relationship between gastric emptying and reflux have yielded conflicting results,[26] a recent study suggests that the rate of proximal stomach emptying may have a more significant effect on reflux. Stacher et al[27] measured gastric emptying of a semisolid meal and performed 24-hour pH-metry in 71 patients with symptoms of both delayed gastric emptying and reflux; they found that slow proximal but not distal gastric emptying correlated with increased 24-hour and postprandial acid exposure.

Helicobacter pylori

It has been suggested that *H. pylori*, known to be a risk factor for peptic ulcer disease and gastric cancer, may protect against GERD because the corpus gastritis caused by this bacteria results in decreased gastric acid production. Conversely, eradication of *H. pylori* has been shown to increase basal gastric acidity and basal gastric acid output.[28] A large epidemiological study found that between 1975 and 1995, hospitalizations for GERD and esophageal adenocarcinoma in the United States rose significantly, whereas those for peptic ulcer disease and gastric cancer fell; the authors hypothesized that the opposing trends for these diseases were due to the declining rate of *Helicobacter pylori* infection in the western population.[29] In another report, Labenz et al[30] described a group of 450 patients with duodenal ulcer who received treatment for *H. pylori* infection; three years after therapy, the incidence of reflux esophagitis was twice as high in the group with successful eradication (26%) compared to those with persistent infection (13%), suggesting again that *H. pylori* may protect against reflux. Subsequent studies found a similar prevalence of *H. pylori* infection for GERD patients and controls; however, the presence of the cagA+ strain of *H. pylori* was protective against more severe forms of GERD, such as Barrett's esophagus.[31-32] More recently an analysis of eight double-blind prospective trials of *H. pylori* therapy in 1165 patients with duodenal ulcer found that eradication of this bacteria does not lead to the development of esophagitis or worsening of symptoms in patients with pre-existing GERD.[33]

Gastroesophageal Junction Factors

Reflux of gastric contents into the esophagus is prevented by two mechanisms at the gastroesophageal junction: (1) the lower esophageal sphincter (LES), a high-pressure zone in the distal esophagus, and (2) the crural diaphragm, which serves to augment the high pressure at the gastroesophageal junction. Failure of one or both of these complementary mechanisms may lead to abnormal esophageal exposure to injurious gastroduodenal contents resulting in esophageal mucosal damage or symptoms of GERD. In mild to moderate nonerosive reflux disease, the basal LES pressure and the crural diaphragm anatomy are frequently normal[34] and many recent studies have established that transient lower esophageal sphincter relaxations (TLESRs) are the major mechanism of reflux in normal subjects and patients with reflux disease.[35-36]

Transient Lower Esophageal Sphincter Relaxations (TLESRs)

Transient lower esophageal relaxations are spontaneous, swallow-independent relaxations of the LES associated with relaxation of the crural diaphragm; they are induced by gastric distention, through a vagally mediated pathway that integrates stimulating and inhibiting factors and, when a threshold of excitation is reached, signals the LES and crural diaphragm to relax. In addition to gastric distention, pharyngeal intubation or stimulation may increase the rate of TLESRs.[37] TLESRs constitute the most common mechanism of reflux in both normal subjects and GERD patients.[35-36] Although TLESRs account for well over 90% or reflux episodes in normal individuals,[35] their contribution to reflux decreases as one moves across the spectrum of disease severity from normal to nonerosive GERD to reflux with endoscopic esophagitis. Thus, in patients with severe disease, in whom hiatal hernias are very common, other mechanisms (such as low basal LES pressure) become increasingly important. A study evaluating the mechanisms responsible for reflux episodes over a 24-hour period in patients with and without hiatal hernia showed that in patients with moderate to large-sized hiatal hernia, the relative contribution of TLESRs to reflux is smaller, with significant amounts of reflux caused by hypotensive LES, swallow-related LES relaxations, deep inspiration, and straining.[38]

Hypotensive LES

Although TLESR is the major mechanism of reflux, a low LES pressure is an important mechanism of reflux in patients with severe GERD. A hypotensive LES (ie, with a basal pressure <10 mm Hg) may allow gastric contents to reflux freely into the esophagus resulting in esophagitis or GERD symptoms. The mechanism by which low LES pressure results in reflux is not completely understood. One possibility is that a combination of a low pressure in LES and hiatus hernia is required for the development of erosive esophagitis. The larger the hernia, the wider the esophageal hiatus, and the more likely that the crural diaphragm component of the sphincter is incompetent.

Although most patients with GERD have a normal LES pressure, a small number, particularly those with severe GERD and erosive esophagitis usually have a low LES pressure. The degree of endoscopic injury appears to correlate with LES pressure. For example, patients with scleroderma who often have severe esophagitis, also have very low LES pressures. Myogenic and neurogenic failure, whether primary or secondary to acid injury, have been proposed as explanations for the low LES pressure, but the mechanism responsible for this has not been well established.[39] Additionally, a low LES pressure can result from external factors, such as gastric distension, foods (chocolate, alcohol), smoking, or medication.

Hiatal Hernia

There are four types of hiatal hernia, the most common of which is a sliding hernia (type I), with a prevalence of 10% to 80% prevalence.[40] Types II, III, and IV are variants of paraesophageal hernias and are less common and together they account for a small percentage of all hiatal hernias.[41] Hiatal hernia is considered significant mainly due to its association with GERD. Most patients with moderate to severe gastroesophageal reflux disease have a type I hiatal hernia.[42] Furthermore, as shown in a study of 66 GERD patients and 16 controls that underwent endoscopy, manometry and pH monitoring, hiatal hernia size correlates with the severity of esophagitis.[43] The herniation of a portion of the stomach into the thoracic cavity can promote reflux in several different ways. Gastric acid present in the hernia sac may easily reflux into the esophagus during swallow-associated relaxations, as the antireflux effect of the crural diaphragm is lost with displacement of the esophagogastric junction. Additionally, patients with hiatal hernia have a lower threshold for triggering of TLESRs elicited by gastric distension.[44] Finally, as explained above, patients with hernia have a higher proportion of reflux resulting from hypotensive LES, swallow-related LES relaxation, deep inspiration and straining.[38] How hiatal hernias develop remains unexplained, but animal[45] and human[46] studies suggest a role for acid-induced esophageal shortening as a possible cause.

Esophageal Factors

Once gastroduodenal contents reach the esophagus, esophageal defense occurs through clearance that empties gastric contents by peristalsis, and neutralization of residual intraluminal acid by means of bicarbonate present in saliva and other secretions.

Esophageal Clearance

Clearance of acid from the esophagus is a two-step process that involves emptying of esophageal refluxate by gravity and peristalsis (primary and/or secondary) followed by neutralization of acid in the esophageal lumen by bicarbonate present in saliva or secreted by esophageal submucosal glands.[47]

Abnormal Peristalsis. Defective primary peristalsis (also known as ineffective esophageal motility) characterized by either absent or low amplitude (<30 mm Hg) contractions in the distal esophagus, can result in impaired esophageal volume clearance.[48] Furthermore, ineffective esophageal motility is the main motility abnormality in GERD patients[49] and peristaltic dysfunction becomes more common as the severity of esophagitis increases, being present in 50% of patients with severe esophagitis.[50] Whether the defective peristalsis seen in GERD patients is a consequence of chronic reflux-related injury or present as a primary smooth muscle abnormality that contributes to the development of GERD is not well understood. Animal models of esophagitis have shown that acute acid injury produces a reduction in LES pressure that is reversible upon resolution of the inflammation.[51-52] However, healing of esophagitis has not resulted in reversion of defects in primary peristalsis in patients with chronic reflux treated with proton pump inhibitors[53] or antireflux surgery.[54] These findings suggest that the defective peristalsis seen in chronic GERD patients constitutes either a primary motility abnormality or an irreversible injury due to chronic exposure to acid.

Acid Neutralization. The second step in esophageal clearance, after emptying of the esophagus through gravity and peristalsis, consists of deacidifying the intraluminal milieu by bicarbonate present mainly in saliva and, to a lesser degree, secreted by the esophageal submucosal glands. Additionally, saliva contains a number of growth factors including epidermal growth factor (EGF), which have the potential to enhance mucosal repair, provide cytoprotection against irritants and decrease the permeability of the esophageal mucosa to hydrogen ions.[55] Conditions in which production of saliva is impaired may lead to defective acid neutralization in the esophagus. For example, prolonged esophageal acid exposure has been shown in patients with chronic xerostomia.[56] Additionally, studies have shown that smoking can contribute to GERD by an anticholinergic effect that decreases production of saliva and results in significant increases in acid clearance time in comparison to nonsmokers.[57]

Epithelial Defense and Repair

Increased exposure to acid, due to a combination of frequent reflux episodes and poor esophageal clearance, can lead to mucosal damage. The esophageal epithelium constitutes a structural barrier to diffusion of acid and pepsin because of tight junctions and an intercellular glycoprotein matrix that, together, result in high epithelial electrical resistance which limits the entry of acid into the tissue. GERD develops when refluxed acidic gastroduodenal contents damage the esophageal intercellular junctions, which then allow easier access for hydrogen ions to come into contact with afferent nerves in the esophageal epithelium which may result in the sensation of heartburn in patients with GERD. Once hydrogen ions enter the cell, phosphates, protein, and carbonic anhydrase-derived bicarbonate act as buffers; when this intracellular buffering capacity is exhausted, esophageal epithelial cells can resort to extrusion of acid by two transmembrane pumps: a Na/H exchanger and a sodium-dependent Cl/HCO_3 exchanger.[5] When the epithelium is finally overwhelmed by an acid load, intracellular pH falls, leading to cell injury, defects in volume regulation, further impairment of the epithelial defense mechanisms with a resulting increase in permeability to acid and, ultimately, cell death and necrosis.[58] Repeated acid exposure may cause continued cell death with subsequent mucosal erosion and endoscopic appearance of erosive GERD. Subsequent to mucosal injury and once high esophageal acid exposure is under control, epithelial repair may be carried out through cell replication and subsequent migration into the injured area.[4]

Summary

The pathophysiology of reflux disease is multifactorial. Pathologic reflux occurs when injurious gastroduodenal contents (acid, pepsin, bile acids) frequently breach the esophagogastric junction because of transient LES relaxations, hypotensive LES, or anatomic disruption (hiatal hernia). After reflux occurs, impaired luminal clearance (peristalsis and acid neutralization) can lead to prolonged exposure to harmful gastroduodenal contents which ultimately overwhelm the epithelial defenses, resulting in symptoms and, in some cases, tissue injury to the esophagus or extraesophageal structures such as the larynx or the lungs.

PATHOPHYSIOLOGY OF EXTRAESOPHAGEAL REFLUX DISEASE

Damage due reflux of gastric contents in the esophagus may extend to supraesophageal structures. The most common extraesophageal manifestations of GERD include pulmonary complaints (ie, chronic cough and wheezing) and ear-nose-throat symptoms (ie, hoarseness, throat clearing, sore throat, and globus).[59,60] Although the factors leading to movement of gastric material from the stomach into the esophagus (ie, gastroesophageal reflux) and the mechanisms of esophageal epithelial injury are understood fairly well, the pathogenetic mechanisms responsible for the extraesophageal presentations of GERD are less clear. The last few years have seen progress in this area, although it is a subject of ongoing debate and active research. What is know about the pathophysiology of lung and laryngeal injury from reflux and the associated symptoms is described below.

Lung Injury due to GERD

A very large case-control study of 92,000 patients with esophagitis compared to 101,000 controls found that having esophagitis increased the risk of pulmonary disease (chronic bronchitis, asthma, chronic obstructive pulmonary disease) by 22 to 55%.[60] Other studies have shown that GERD is present in 50 to 80% of asthmatic patients.[61–64] That said, it is important to keep in mind that the relationship between gastroesophageal reflux and pulmonary disease is bidirectional. In other words, although reflux may cause cough or worsen asthma, cough and asthma can induce reflux be changing the pressure differences between the abdominal and thoracic cavities. In addition to the negative intrathoracic pressure produced by coughing or during an asthma attack, some asthma medications can decrease the tone of the lower esophageal sphincter, which can also promote reflux.[65,66] Thus, establishing a clear cause-and-effect relationship between GERD and asthma is difficult because either condition may induce the other. This notion is further supported by the fact that whereas more than half of asthmatic patients experience typical reflux symptoms,[67] other asthmatics may have significant GERD in the absence of classic reflux symptoms such as heartburn or regurgitation. A study by Irwin and collaborators[68] reported that clinically silent GERD may occur in nearly 24% of asthmatics.

Potential injurious agents involved in GERD-related lung disease include a mixture both gastric (acid and pepsin) as well as duodenal contents (bile acids and the pancreatic enzyme trypsin).[69] Reflux of these agents into the esophagus or beyond can cause cough or an asthmatic response by the vagally mediated esophagotracheobronchial cough reflex, or by direct injury as a consequence of mucosal contact, either macro or microaspiration (Color Plate 2).[63,64,70,71]

The tracheobronchial reflex, although not fully elucidated, likely involves a complex reflex arc beginning with the stimulation of sensory nerves in the esophagus. The exact role of refluxate in triggering cough by means of this reflex is the subject of debate and ongoing research, but from an evolutionary standpoint it can be speculated that a distal esophageal-bronchial reflex evolved as a mechanism designed to protect the lungs from aspiration of gastric contents.[72] The vagally mediated cough reflex was supported by a study using distal esophageal acid perfusion compared to saline. There was a significant increase in cough frequency in the acid group compared with the saline group. When the afferent pathway was blocked by the instillation of lidocaine, there was a decrease in the frequency of acid-induced cough. Blocking the efferent pathway with nebulized ipratropium bromide also inhibited cough, an effect not seen with esophageal ipratropium.[73]

Ing et al[74] studied 13 patients with chronic persistent cough that was unexplained after a standard diagnostic assessment; these patients were compared to 9 healthy controls matched for age, lung function, and body mass index. Twenty-four hour ambulatory oesophageal pH monitoring revealed a significantly higher number of acid reflux episodes and increased esophageal acid exposure in the patients. In patients, cough occurred simultaneously with many reflux episodes. However, they also noted the occurrence of cough within 5 minutes following reflux and, conversely, reflux following cough. They theorized that a self-perpetuating mechanism may exist whereby acid reflux causes cough via the esophagotracheobronchial reflex, and the cough, in turn, amplifies reflux via increased negative intrathoracic pressure. In a later study, Irwin et al[72] suggested that the presence of acid is not always required to elicit cough through a reflux-induced reflex arc. They studied eight patients with cough thought to be due to reflux. All patients had persistent cough despite acid suppression and normalization of pH-metry after medical therapy. Antireflux surgery resulted in clinical improvement of cough, suggesting a role for deacidifed reflux material as a trigger for cough. This notion has recently gained further support based upon impedance-pH monitoring that enables measurement of non-acid reflux, as explained later on.

Microaspiration and macroaspiration from proximal esophageal reflux are the other proposed mechanisms for GERD-induced cough. Studies evaluating the effect of airway acidification on bronchoconstriction describe acid-induced activation of a subpopulation of primary sensory neurons in the airway, the so-called capsaicin-sensitive primary sensory neurons, which may release several different neuropeptides such as substance P and neurokinin A.[75] These neuropeptides can stimulate bronchial smooth muscle leading to bronchoconstriction. Whether nonacid reflux can activate the same pathway is not known. As mentioned earlier, the presence of acid in refluxed material is not always required to elicit cough.[73] Conventional pH monitoring is not adequate for the detection of reflux with a pH above 4.0, that is, nonacid reflux. Combined multichannel intraluminal impedance and pH (MII-pH) monitoring, a newer technique for reflux monitoring, has the ability to identify all types of reflux and to evaluate symptom associations with both nonacid and acid reflux. This technique has been recently used to study the role of nonacid reflux as a cause for cough. It is important to recognize that acid suppressive therapy only changes the chemical composition of the gastroesophageal refluxate, but it does not actually stop reflux from occurring. Therefore, microaspiration of nonacid materials or stimulation of the esophagotracheobronchial reflex by nonacid reflux may both continue to occur in the presence of pharmacologic acid suppression.

In a recent study, Sifrim et al[76] reported on the relationship between nonacid reflux and cough in 22 patients. They found that the majority of cough episodes (70%) occurred "independent" of reflux, but 30% of cough episodes were temporally associated with reflux. In half of these cases (51%), cough preceded reflux, whereas in the other half cough was preceded by acid reflux (32%) or nonacid reflux (17%). It is, however, important to recognize that these studies were performed "off therapy." Studies in patients on therapy generally show a larger proportion of nonacid reflux episodes, which is to be expected following pharmacologic buffering of the gastric contents. Tutuian recently showed that up to a quarter of patients with chronic cough persisting despite acid-suppressive therapy have a temporal association between cough and nonacid reflux.[77] This study also described the effects of fundoplication in six patients with persistent cough despite proton-pump inhibitors in whom ambulatory MII-pH revealed a positive association between nonacid reflux and cough. Following antireflux surgery, all six patients remained asymptomatic and off acid suppression when followed for a median 17 months (range 12 to 27 months). This study lacked a control arm and was based on subjective endpoints (symptoms), without quantification of reflux after the therapeutic intervention. Therefore, this information is important and encouraging, but it should be regarded as "hypothesis-generating" information that awaits confirmation by larger, randomized controlled trials.

In summary, GERD is often included in the differential diagnosis for patients presenting with pulmonary complaints such as chronic cough or asthma. Reflux may lead to these clinical presentations by the esophagotracheobronchial reflex, or through macro or microaspiration resulting in direct mucosal injury. However, the relationship between gastroesophageal reflux and pulmonary disease is complex and its study is challenging because of the two-way causality: reflux can lead to cough and asthma, and these conditions may in turn induce reflux by increasing intrathoracic negative pressure. Furthermore, patients with pulmonary disease caused by reflux may or may not present with the typical symptoms of heartburn and regurgitation. Finally, recent data suggest that failure of acid suppressing medications to improve cough or asthma may not always rule out reflux as a cause for pulmonary symptoms. In some patients with persistent symptoms despite acid suppression, nonacid reflux may be a culprit that is now measurable by impedance-pH monitoring. For these patients, a different therapeutic approach such as fundoplication may be considered, but further research is needed in this area.

Laryngeal Injury due to GERD

Laryngopharyngeal reflux (LPR) is the retrograde movement of gastric refluxate into the laryngopharynx. Common symptoms attributed to LPR are hoarseness, throat clearing, cough, and globus pharyngeus. Common laryngoscopic findings of LPR include laryngeal hyperemia and edema, granuloma, cobblestoning of the posterior pharynx, and laryngeal polyps. In some studies, up to 60% of chronic laryngitis and sore throat may be related to GERD, and up to 15% of patients present to ENT physicians with GERD-related complaints.[78,79] On the other hand, it is very important to keep in mind that the symptoms and signs of LPR are not very specific and can be the result of injury through non-GERD mechanisms, making the study of the pathophysiology of LPR and related symptoms challenging.

LPR may cause symptoms by direct and indirect mechanisms (see Color Plate 2), though the exact pathogenesis remains a controversial issue. The direct mechanism involves irritation of laryngeal mucosa by the gastric refluxate (HCl, pepsin), and much of our knowledge of this mechanism has been derived from animal models. Delahunty and Cherry[80] showed that the application of gastric juice to a dog's vocal folds caused the formation of granulomas. Adhami et al[81] evaluated the role of gastric and duodenal contents on injury of different laryngeal structures in dogs. They concluded that pepsin and conjugated bile acids were responsible for laryngeal tissue injury, and the vocal folds were the most sensitive laryngeal structure to acid-related injury. Duodenal refluxate (unconjugated bile acids and trypsin) did not cause laryngeal issue. Caustic refluxate may also impair the ciliated respiratory epithelium of the larynx, which normally clears mucus from the airways. This may account for the excessive throat clearing seen in LPR patients.[82]

Although gastroesophageal reflux disease (GERD) and LPR are related, it must be noted that the pathophysiology of these two diseases is different. When compared to the esophageal mucosa, the laryngeal mucosa is more susceptible to injury, which may be caused by much lower levels of acid and pepsin exposure when compared to the esophageal epithelium. One of the carbonic anhydrase isoenzymes, CA III, has been shown to have increased expression in the esophageal mucosa in response to refluxate exposure, but is depleted in the laryngeal mucosa after acid exposure. It is also believed that laryngeal mucosal damage is much less reversible than esophageal mucosal damage due to a thinner and less adaptive epithelium in the larynx.[83,84]

There may be a mechanism by which acid affects laryngeal mucosa through a local H+/K+ ATPase similar to that seen in gastric parietal cells. A pilot study performed by Altman et al[85] using immunohistochemical staining with monoclonal antibodies for both the alpha and beta subunits of the H+/K+ ATPase found strong staining in the serous cells and ducts of the minor seromucinous glands in the larynx of two cadaveric specimens. There was no staining in normal gastric cells unless they were parietal cells. This study raises the possibility the LPR patients may have higher levels of acid due to a functional H+/K+ ATPase in the larynx.

It has been suggested that sensory deficits may play a prominent role in LPR. The larynx is densely innervated, and any abnormal reflux normally elicits a protective cough; failure of this reflex may permit greater exposure to noxious agents and ultimately lead to tissue damage and the associated LPR symptoms. The possibility of a failed sensory mechanism causing LPR was illustrated in a study by Aviv et al,[86] who found decreased laryngeal adductor reflexes in response to endoscopic administration of air-puff stimuli in LPR patients.

Similar to the model for reflux leading to pulmonary disease, gastroesophageal reflux may induce laryngeal complications not only by direct mucosal contact, but also through a reflex mechanism. Shaker et al[87] investigated a possible esophagoglottal closure reflex using concurrent videoendoscopy and manometry to assess glottal and upper esophageal sphincter (UES) responses to esophageal distention by air and balloon distention. They concluded that esophageal distention by either air or a balloon evokes a glottal closure mechanism, and that this reflex is elicited most easily by distention of the proximal esophagus. This esophagoglottal closure reflex may play an important role in preventing LPR. Another potential indirect mechanism of laryngeal damage secondary to reflux is thought to involve irritation of the distal esophagus that stimulates a vagally mediated response of bronchoconstriction. This reflex arc may account for the chronic cough which in turn can irritate the laryngoparhyngeal structures. These vagal afferents may also cause a transient decrease in UES pressure, which could theoretically facilitate movement of refluxed material into the supraesophageal structures. The exact reason for UES relaxation remains incompletely understood and studies addressing this issue have yielded variable results. Vakil et al,[88] in a study with normal volunteers and patients with esophagitis, showed that the upper esophageal sphincter exhibited normal basal pressure in patients with esophagitis and that esophageal acid exposure, either spontaneous or experimental, does not affect UES pressure in normal volunteers or in patients with esophagitis. In a study using a cylindrical balloon to distend the proximal esophagus, Kahrilas et al[89] showed that the rapidity and spatial pattern of esophageal distention, rather than discrimination of the type of material causing the distension, determines whether or not UES relaxation occurs. It is evident that the exact role of the UES in LPR remains incompletely defined. One hopes further research in this area will clarify this issue.

Another important question is whether increased esophageal acid exposure correlates with LPR. Using ambulatory 24-h esophageal pH monitoring, abnormal esophageal acid exposure is found in 55 to 79% of patients with chronic hoarseness.[90] In a study of ENT patients with suspected GERD whose symptoms improved with aggressive acid-suppressive therapy, three important laryngeal sites —the posterior pharyngeal wall, true vocal folds, and arytenoid medial wall—showed significantly more injury than in healthy subjects.[91] This suggests that, at least in some patients, reducing reflux (objectively quantified as normalization of esophageal acid exposure) can lead to improvement of LPR symptoms. This supported not only symptomatic but also laryngeal improvements of the signs on aggressive acid suppression (PPIs twice daily for 4 months).[79] However, it is important to remember that not all patients with increased esophageal acid exposure develop LPR, and that some patients with symptoms and sings suggestive of LPR may have injury due to nonreflux causes or may have a multifactorial laryngeal injury.

There is a subgroup of patients whose LPR symptoms will not respond to aggressive acid suppression therapy, and it may be difficult clinically to assess whether or not reflux is playing a role in their symptoms. Until recently, these patients may have been told that reflux could be excluded as a cause of their symptoms if they did not respond to PPI therapy. Combined multichannel intraluminal impedance-pH (MII-pH) testing allows for the identification of nonacid reflux and its association with laryngeal symptoms. However, symptom association studies to assess the temporal relationship between reflux episodes and symptoms are more difficult to perform when dealing with symptoms of long duration (hoarseness, for instance) as opposed to short episodic presentations (such as cough or heartburn). Nonetheless, MII-pH studies have shown that in some patients with LPR, nonacid reflux could potentially be a culprit. Mainie et al[92] used a telephone interview to evaluate the effect of Nissen fundoplication in 18 patients with symptomatic reflux (9 with typical symptoms) documented by impedance-pH on PPI BID. Symptoms were due to nonacid reflux in 14, and acid reflux in 4 patients. After a mean follow-up of 14 months in 17 available patients, all but one was asymptomatic or markedly improved. Three of these patients suffered from laryngeal symptoms and were among the symptom-free patients on follow-up. Although surgical fundoplication may be beneficial in these patients, it should be stressed that, similar to the experience in treating nonacid-related cough, this study was uncontrolled and based on subjective outcomes, without quantification of reflux after surgery. These results are contrasted with a controlled study of 10 patients who underwent fundoplication for suspected laryngopharyngeal reflux that had not responded to a twice-daily PPI.[93] Although there was no randomization, when fundoplication subjects were compared to 15 controls that remained on medication but did not undergo surgery, fundoplication offered no advantage for relief of laryngeal symptoms. However, it must be pointed out that the decision to perform surgery was based solely on refractoriness to PPI, without documentation that the ongoing symptoms were due to reflux.

In summary, laryngeal injury and the associated laryngeal symptoms may be caused by reflux disease, either by direct mucosal contact or by a reflex pathway. The laryngeal epithelium appears to be more susceptible to damage from reflux compared to the esophageal epithelium, and controlling acid reflux does not always result in clinical improvement. Early and limited data suggest a possible for role for nonacid reflux in some patients with persistent symptoms despite acid suppression, but large controlled trials will be required to confirm this. It is very important to remember that there aren't any laryngeal symptoms or exam findings that are unique to or specific to reflux as a cause, and other potential etiologies may be involved, acting either alone or in concert with reflux.

REFERENCES

1. Locke GR, Talley NJ, Fett SL, Zinmeister AR, Melton LJ. Prevalence and clinical spectrum of gastroesophageal reflux: a population-based study in Olmsted County, Minnesota. *Gastroenterology.* 1997;112:1448–1456.
2. Vaezi MF, Singh S, Richter JE. Role of acid and duodenogastric reflux in esophageal mucosal injury: a review of animal and human studies. *Gastroenterology.* 1995; 108:1897–1907.

3. Goldberg HI, Dodds WJ, Gee S, et al. Role of acid and pepsin in acute experimental esophagitis. *Gastroenterology.* 1969; 56(2):223-230.
4. Orlando RC. Pathogenesis of gastroesophageal disease. *Gastroenterol Clin North Am.* 2002;31:S35-S44.
5. Orlando RC. Pathophysiology of gastroesophageal reflux disease: offensive factors and tissue resistance. In: Orlando RC, ed. *Gastroesophageal Reflux Disease.* New York, NY: Marcel Dekker; 2000:165-192.
6. Tuttle SG, Ruffin F, Bettarello A. The physiology of heartburn. *Ann Intern Med.* 1961;55:292.
7. Gillen P, Keeling P, Byrne PJ, et al. Barrett's esophagus: pH profile. *Br J Surg.* 1987;74:774-776.
8. Hennessy TPJ. Barrett's esophagus. *Br J Surg.* 1985;72:336-340.
9. Stein HJ, Siewert JR. Barrett's esophagus: pathogenesis, epidemiology, functional abnormalities, malignant degeneration, and surgical management. *Dysphagia.* 1993;8:276-288.
10. Stein HJ, Barlow AP, DeMeester TR, et al. Complications of gastroesophageal reflux disease. *Ann Surg.* 1992;216:35-43.
11. Zamost BJ, Hirschberg J, Ippoliti AF. Esophagitis in scleroderma: prevalence and risk factors. *Gastroenterology.* 1987; 92:421-428.
12. Hirschowitz BI. A critical analysis, with appropriate controls, of gastric acid and pepsin secretion in clinical esophagitis. *Gastroenterology.* 1991;101:1149-1158.
13. Miller LS, Vinayek R, Frucht H, et al. Reflux esophagitis in patients with Zollinger Ellison syndrome. *Gastroenterology.* 1990;98:341-346.
14. Cross FS, Wangesteen OH. Role of bile and pancreatic juice in the production of esophageal erosions and anemia. *Proc Soc Exp Biol Med.* 1961;77:862-866.
15. Gillison EW, DeCastro VAM, Nyhus LM, et al. The significance of bile in reflux esophagitis. *Surg Gynecol Obstet.* 1972: 134:419-424.
16. Harmon JW, Johnson LF, Maydonovitch CL. Effects of acid and bile salts on the rabbit esophageal mucosa. *Dig Dis Sci.* 1981;26:65-72.
17. Kivilaakso E, Fromm D, Silen W. Effect of bile salts and related compounds on isolated esophageal mucosa. *Surgery.* 1980; 87:280-285.
18. Moffat RC, Berkas EM. Bile esophagitis. *Arch Surg.* 1965;91:963-966.
19. Vaezi MF. Duodenogastric reflux. In: Castell DO, Richter JE, eds. *The Esophagus.* 3rd ed. Philadelphia, Pa: Lippincott Williams & Wilkins; 1999:421-436.
20. Vaezi MF, Richter JE. Role of acid and duodenogastroesophageal reflux in gastroesophageal reflux disease. *Gastroenterology.* 1996;111:1192-1199.
21. Marshall RFK, Anggiansah A, Owen WA, Owen WJ. The relationship between acid and bile reflux and symptoms in gastroesophageal reflux disease. *Gut.* 1997;40: 182-187.
22. Sears RJ, Champion G, Richter JE. Characteristics of partial gastrectomy (PG) patients with esophageal symptoms of doudenogastric reflux. *Am J Gastroenterol.* 1995;90:211-215.
23. Vaezi MF, Sears R, Richter JE. Placebo-controlled trial of cisapride in postgastrectomy patients with duodenogastric reflux. *Dig Dis Sci.* 1996;41:754-763.
24. Koek G, Sifrim D, Degreef T, Janssens J, Tack J. The GABA B agonist baclofen reduces duodeno-gastro-esophageal reflux (DGER) and symptoms in patients with reflux disease refractory to proton pump inhibitor therapy. *Gastroenterology.* 2001:120:A34.
25. Vela MF, Camacho-Lobato L, Srinivasan R, Tutuian R, Katz PO, Castell DO. Intraesophageal impedance and pH measurement of acid and nonacid reflux: effect of omeprazole. *Gastroenterology.* 2001; 120:1599-1606.
26. Richter JE. Do we know the cause of reflux disease? *Eur J Gastroenterol Hepatol.* 1999;11:S3-S9.

27. Stacher G, Lenglinger J, Bergman H, et al. Gastric emptying: a contributory factor in gastro-oesophageal reflux activity? *Gut.* 2000;47:661-666.
28. Feldman M, Cryer B, Lee E. Effects of Helicobacter pylori gastritis on gastric secretion in healthy human beings. *Am J Physiol.* 1998;274(6 pt 1):G1011-G1017.
29. El-Serag HB, Sonnenberg A. Opposing trends of peptic ulcer and reflux disease. *Gut.* 1998;43:327-333.
30. Labenz J, Blum AL, Bayerdorffer E, at al. Curing Helicobacter pylori infection in patients with duodenal ulcer may provoke reflux esophagitis. *Gastroenterology.* 1997;112:1442-1447.
31. Vicari J, Peek R, Falk G, et al. The seroprevalence of cagA-positive Helicobacter pylori strains in the spectrum of gastroesophageal disease. *Gastroenterology.* 1998;115:50-57.
32. Vaezi M, Falk G, Peek R. CagA-positive strains of Helicobacter pylori may protect against Barrett's esophagus. *Am J Gastroenterol.* 2000;2206:2206-2211.
33. Laine L, Sugg J. Effect of Helicobacter pylori eradication on development of erosive esophagitis and gastroesophageal reflux disease symptoms: a post hoc analysis of eight double blind prospective studies. *Am J Gastroenterol.* 2002;97:2992-2997.
34. Mittal RK, Chowdry NK, Liu J. Is the sphincter function of crural diaphragm impaired in patients with reflux esophagitis? *Gastroenterology.* 1995;108:A169.
35. Dodds WJ, Dent J, Hogan WJ, et al. Mechanisms of gatroesophageal reflux in patients with reflux esophagitis. *N Engl J Med.* 1982;307:1547-1552.
36. Mittal RK, Holloway RH, Penagini R, Blakshaw LA, Dent J. Transient lower esophageal relaxation. *Gastroenterology.* 1995;109:601-610.
37. Mittal RK, Chiareli C, Liu J, Shaker R. Characteristics of LES relaxation induced stimulation of the pharynx with minute amounts of water. *Gastroenterology.* 1996;111:378-384.
38. Van Herwaarden MA, Samsom M, Smouth AJPM. Excess gastroesophageal reflux in patients with hiatus hernia is caused by mechanisms other than transient LES relaxations. *Gastroenterology.* 2000;119: 1439-1446.
39. Mittal R. Pathophysiology of gastroesophageal reflux disease: motility factors. In: Castell DO, Richter JE, eds. *The Esophagus.* 3rd ed. Philadelphia, Pa: Lippincott Williams & Wilkins; 1999:397-408.
40. Skinner DB. Hernias. In: Berk JE, ed. *Gastroenterology.* 4th ed. Philadelphia, Pa: WB Saunders; 1985:705.
41. Peridikis G, Hinder RA. Paraesophageal hiatal hernia. In: Nyhus LM, Condon RE, eds. *Hernia.* Philadelphia, Pa: JB Lippincott Co; 1995:544.
42. Mittal R, Balaban R. The esophagogastric junction. *N Engl J Med.* 1997;336: 924-932.
43. Jones MP, Sloan SS, Rabine JC, et al. Hiatal hernia size is the dominant determinant of esophagitis presence and severity in gastroesophageal reflux disease. *Am J Gastroenterol.* 2001;96:1711-1717.
44. Kharilas PJ, Shi G, Manka M, Hoehl R. Increased frequency of transient lower esophageal relaxation induced by gastric distension in reflux patients with hiatal hernia. *Gastroenterology.* 2000;118: 688-695.
45. White R, Zhang Y, Morris G, Paterson WG. Esophagitis-related esophageal shortening in opossum is associated with longitudinal muscle hyperresponsiveness. *Am J Physiol Gastrointest Liver Physiol.* 2001; 280:G463-G469.
46. Dunne DP, Paterson WG. Acid-induced esophageal shortening in humans: a cause of hiatus hernia? *Can J Gastroenterol.* 2000;14:847-850.
47. Helms JF, Dodds WJ, Pelc LR, et al. Effect of esophageal emptying and saliva on clearance of acid from the esophagus. *N Engl J Med.* 1984;310:284-288.
48. Kahrilas PJ, Dodds WJ, Hogan WJ. Effect of peristaltic dysfunction on esophageal

volume clearance. *Gastroenterology.* 1988;94:73-80.

49. Fouad YM, Katz PO, Hatlebakk JG, Castell DO. Ineffective esophageal motility: the most common motility abnormality in patients with GERD-associated respiratory symptoms. *Am J Gastroenterol.* 1999;94: 1464-1467.
50. Kahrilas PJ, Dodds WJ, Hogan WJ, et al. Esophageal peristaltic dysfunction in peptic esophagitis. *Gastroenterology.* 1986; 91:897-904.
51. Eastwood GL, Castell DO, Higgs RH. Experimental esophagitis in cats impairs lower esophageal sphincter pressure. *Gastroenterology.* 1975;69:146-153.
52. Higgs RH, Castell DO, Eastwood GL. Studies on the mechanism of esophagitis-induced lower esophageal sphincter hypotension in cats. *Gastroenterology.* 1976;71:51-57.
53. Timmer R, Breumelhof R, Nadorp JH, Smout AJ. Oesophageal motility and gastro-oesophageal reflux before and after healing of reflux esophagitis. A study using 24-hour ambulatory pH and pressure monitoring. *Gut.* 1994;35:1519-1522.
54. Rydberg L, Ruth M, Lundell L. Does esophageal motor function improve with time after successful antireflux surgery? Results of a prospective, randomized clinical study. *Gut.* 1997;41:82-86.
55. Sarosiek J, Feng T, McCallum R. The interrelationship between salivary epidermal growth factor and the functional integrity of the esophageal mucosa. *Am J Med Sci.* 1991;302:359-362.
56. Korsten MA, Rosman AS, Fishbein S, et al. Chronic xerostomia increases esophageal acid exposure and is associated with esophageal injury. *Am J Med.* 1991;90: 701-706.
57. Kharilas PJ, Gupta RR. The effect of cigarette smoking and salivation on esophageal acid clearance. *J Lab Clin Med.* 1989;114:431-438.
58. Orlando RC. Pathophysiology of gastroesophageal reflux disease: esophageal epithelial resistance. In: Castell DO, Richter JE, eds. *The Esophagus.* Philadelphia, Pa: Lippincott; 1999:409-419.
59. Fontana, GA, Pistolesi, M. Chronic cough and gastrooesophageal reflux. *Thorax.* 2003;58:1092-1095.
60. El-Serag HB, Sonnenberg A. Comorbid occurrence of laryngeal or pulmonary disease with esophagitis in United States military veterans. *Gastroenterology.* 1997; 113:755-760.
61. Harding, SM, Richter, JE, Guzzo, MR, et al. Asthma and gastroesophageal reflux: acid suppressive therapy improves asthma outcome. *Am J Med.* 1996;100:395-405.
62. Mays EE. Intrinsic asthma in adults. Association with gastroesophageal reflux. *JAMA.* 1976;236:2626-2628.
63. Sontag SJ, O'Connell S, Khandelwal S, et al. Most asthmatics have gastroesophageal reflux with or without bronchodilator therapy. *Gastroenterology.* 1990; 99:613-620.
64. Vaezi MF. Extraesophageal manifestations of gastroesophageal reflux disease. *Clin Cornerstone.* 2003;5:32-38.
65. Sontag SJ, O'Connell S, Khandelwal S, et al. Effect of positions, eating, and bronchodilators on gastroesophageal reflux in asthmatics. *Dig Dis Sci.* 1990;35:849-856.
66. Simpson WG. Gastroesophageal reflux disease and asthma. Diagnosis and management. *Arch Intern Med.* 1995;155: 798-803.
67. Field SK, Underwood M, Brant R, Cowie RL. Prevalence of gastroesophageal reflux symptoms in asthma. *Chest.* 1996;109: 316-322.
68. Irwin RS, Curley FJ, French CL. Difficult-to-control asthma. Contributing factors and outcome of a systematic management protocol. *Chest.* 1993;103:1662-1669.
69. Vaezi MF. Therapy insight: gastroesophageal reflux disease and laryngopharyngeal reflux. *Nat Clin Pract Gastroenterol Hepatol.* 2005;2:595-603.
70. Groen JN, Smout AJ. Supra-oesophageal manifestations of gastro-oesophageal re-

flux disease. *Eur J Gastroenterol Hepatol.* 2003;15:1339-1350.
71. Barish CF, Wu WC, Castell DO. Respiratory complications of gastro-oesophageal reflux. *Arch Intern Med.* 1985;145: 1882-1888.
72. Irwin RS, Madison JM, Fraire AE. The cough reflex and its relation to gastro-oesophageal reflux. *Am J Med.* 2000; 108(suppl 4a):73S-78S.
73. Irwin RS, Zawacki JK, Wilson M, et al. Chronic cough due to gastro-oesophageal reflux disease: failure to resolve despite total/near-total elimination of esophageal acid. *Chest.* 2002;121:1132-1140.
74. Ing AJ, Ngu MC, Breslin AB. Chronic persistent cough and gastro-oesophageal reflux. *Thorax.* 1991;46:479-483.
75. Ricciardolo FL. Mechanisms of citric acid-induced bronchoconstriction. *Am J Med.* 2001;111(8A):18S-24S.
76. Sifrim, D, Dupont, L, Blondeau, K, et al. Weakly acidic reflux in patients with chronic unexplained cough during 24 hour pressure, pH, and impedance monitoring. *Gut.* 2005;54:449-454.
77. Tutuian, R, Mainie, I, Agrawal, A, Adams, D, Castell, DO. Nonacid reflux in patients with chronic cough on acid-suppressive therapy. *Chest.* 2006;130:386-391.
78. Vaezi MF, Hicks DM, Abelson TI, Richter JE. Laryngeal signs and symptoms and gastroesophageal reflux disease (GERD): a critical assessment of cause and effect association. *Clin Gastroenterol Hepatol.* 2003;1:333-344.
79. Qadeer MA, Swoger J, Milstein C, et al. Correlation between symptoms and laryngeal signs in laryngopharyngeal reflux. *Laryngoscope.* 2005;115:1947-1952.
80. Delahunty JE, Cherry J. Experimentally produced vocal cord granulomas. *Laryngoscope.* 1968;78:1937-1940.
81. Adhami T, Goldblum JR, Richter JE, Vaezi MF. The role of gastric and duodenal agents in laryngeal injury: an experimental canine model. *Am J Gastroenterol.* 2004;99:2098-2106.
82. Hanson DG, Jiang JJ. Diagnosis and management of chronic laryngitis associated with reflux. *Am J Med.* 2000;108: 112S-119S.
83. Axford SE, Sharp N, Ross PE, et al. Cell biology of laryngeal epithelial defenses in health and disease: preliminary studies. *Ann Otol Rhinol Laryngol.* 2001; 110:1099-1108.
84. Johnston N, Bulmer D, Gill GA, et al. Cell biology of laryngeal epithelial defenses in health and disease: further studies. *Ann Otol Rhinol Laryngol.* 2003;112:481-491.
85. Altman KW, Haines GK 3rd, Hammer ND, Radosevich JA. The H+/K+ ATPase (proton) pump is expressed in human laryngeal submucosal glands. *Laryngoscope.* 2003;113:1927-1930.
86. Aviv JE, Lui H, Parides M, Kaplan ST, Close LG. Laryngopharyngeal sensory deficits in patients with laryngopharyngeal reflux and dysphagia. *Ann Otol Rhinol Laryngol.* 2000;109:1000-1006.
87. Shaker R, Dodds WJ, Ren J, Hogan WJ, Arndorfer RC. Esophagoglottal closure reflex: a mechanism of airway protection. *Gastroenterology.* 1992;102:857-861.
88. Vakil NB, Kahrilas PJ, Dodds WJ, Vanagunas A. Absence of an upper esophageal sphincter response to acid reflux. *Am J Gastroenterol.* 1989;84:606-610.
89. Kahrilas PJ, Dodds WJ, Dent J, Wyman JB, Hogan WJ, Arndorfer RC. Upper esophageal sphincter function during belching. *Gastroenterology.* 1986;91:133-140.
90. Richter JE. Typical and atypical presentations of gastroesophageal reflux disease: The role of esophageal testing in diagnosis and management. *Gastroenterol Clin North Am.* 1996;25:75-102.
91. Vaezi MF. Are there specific laryngeal signs for gastroesophageal reflux disease? *Gastroenterology.* 2000;118:2639.
92. Mainie I, Tutuian R, Agrawal A, Adams D, Castell DO. Combined multichannel intraluminal impedance-pH monitoring to select patients with persistent gastro-oesophageal reflux for laparoscopic

Nissen fundoplication. *Br J Surg.* 2006; 93:1483-1487.
93. Swoger J, Ponsky J, Hicks D, et al. Surgical fundoplication for laryngopharyngeal reflux unresponsive to aggressive acid suppression: a controlled study. *Clin Gastroenterol Hepatol.* 2006;4:433-441.

3

Laryngitis: From the Gastroenterologist's Point of View

Michael F. Vaezi

Chronic laryngeal signs and symptoms associated with GERD are often referred to as reflux laryngitis or laryngopharyngeal reflux (LPR). It is estimated that up to 15% of all visits to the otolaryngology offices are because of manifestations of LPR. Injury may occur as a result of one or chronic reflux of gastroduodenal contents directly injuring the laryngeal mucosa. The diagnosis of LPR is usually made on the basis of presenting symptoms and associated laryngeal signs including laryngeal edema and erythema. However, the laryngeal findings in LPR are nonspecific leading to overdiagnosis of this condition in many. Current recommendation for management for of this group of patients is empiric therapy with twice daily PPIs for 1 to 2 months. In majority of those who are unresponsive to such therapy other causes of laryngeal irritation are considered. Surgical fundoplication is most effective in those who are responsive to acid suppressive therapy.

INTRODUCTION

Gastroesophageal reflux disease (GERD) is implicated in many patients with chronic laryngitis. Ear, nose, and throat (ENT) physicians often refer to this condition as Laryngopharyngeal reflux (LPR) representing the retrograde movement of gastric contents, including acid, pepsin as well as bile acids, into the laryngopharynx.[1,2] Typical LPR symptoms include dysphonia, globus pharyngeus (sensation of lump in throat), mild dysphagia, chronic cough, and nonproductive throat clearing (Table 3-1).

The controversy in diagnosis and treatment of LPR patients stems from lack of a gold standard diagnostic modality. This has led to overdiagnosis of LPR resulting in unnecessary diagnostic testing and treatment for a group of patients whose symptoms may not be from GERD. The main driving force of LPR diagnosis appears to be laryngoscopic findings in

Table 3–1. Symptoms Attributed to Laryngopharyngeal Reflux

• Hoarseness
• Dysphonia
• Sore or burning throat
• Excessive throat clearing
• Chronic cough
• Globus pharyngeus
• Dysphagia
• Postnasal drip
• Laryngospasm

a symptomatic patient with throat symptoms. However, there are no identifiable laryngeal signs which can implicate GERD as the definitive cause for patients' symptoms and laryngeal irritations. One study of 105 normal, healthy, adults revealed at least one finding associated with reflux during laryngoscopy in 86% of healthy volunteers without any throat symptoms; highlighting the nonspecific nature of the laryngeal findings currently attributed to GERD.[3] In a meta-analysis which reviewed the data of pH probe readings in patients with LPR and in controls, 10 to 60% of the control patients demonstrated reflux.[4] Studies such as these reveal that the "LPR" may be overdiagnosed in many patients.

In this chapter we highlight the current knowledge and controversy in LPR from a gastroenterologist point of view.

PATHOPHYSIOLOGY

The two predominant pathophysiologic mechanisms for LPR accepted by most experts are direct or indirect laryngeal exposure to various injurious contents of the stomach. The direct mechanism simply results from the actions of caustic gastric contents such as acid, pepsin and/or bile acids interacting with mucosa in the laryngopharynx. The indirect mechanism is thought to result from reflux material interacting with structures more distal to the larynx. It is thought that this irritation evokes a vagally mediated response of bronchoconstriction; possibly causing the commonly associated nonproductive cough.[4] In LPR the former mechanism may be more important.

The specific agent(s) responsible for producing ENT symptoms and laryngeal pathology including laryngitis, vocal fold lesions, and even laryngeal carcinoma are currently unknown and the subject of many debates. Potential candidates include gastric contents, acid and pepsin, and duodenal contents, both bile acids and the pancreatic enzyme trypsin. Previous animal studies suggested injurious potential for both acid and pepsin, reporting a significant role for both agents in causing laryngeal lesions.[5] A recent study extended the above observations and showed that the bile constituents, conjugated and unconjuated bile acids as well as trypsin, at different pH values (pH 1-7) caused no histologic laryngeal injury in a dog model.[6] The most injurious agents were acid and pepsin in an acidic pH. This finding highlights the importance of acidic refluxate in causing laryngeal inflammation and casts doubt on the significance of bile constituents in this region. This finding is clinically important since some reports implicate the reflux of nonacidic duodenal contents as the cause of persistent laryngitis in patients unresponsive to aggressive acid suppression.

In humans, it is difficult to isolate the injurious potential of each of the above listed agents, mainly because the gastric milieu refluxing into the esophagus is commonly a mixture of gastric and duodenal contents. Although laryngeal injury may occur with intermittent acid/pepsin exposure in animals, this area is not well studied in humans and is subject to controversy. The advent of impedance/pH monitoring as the indirect marker for the reflux of gastroduodenal contents may shed some important light into the possible contribution of acid and nonacid reflux in patients with LPR who continue to be symptomatic despite acid suppressive therapy.

CLINICAL MANIFESTATIONS

Most patients diagnosed with LPR may not have the classic symptoms of GERD. One series of patients with otolaryngologic symptoms who were found to have LPR complained of the following symptoms: dysphonia (71%), cough (51%), globus pharyngeus (47%), throat clearing (42%), and dysphagia (35%).[7] These symptoms were often intermittent. Additionally, heartburn and regurgitation which are hallmark symptoms suggesting the presence of GERD were not present in most these patients. It is estimated that up to 50% of patients with laryngeal and voice disorders have reflux.[8]

In patients suspected with LPR various laryngeal signs are attributed to GERD such as erythema, edema, pseudosulcus, ventricular obliteration, and postcricoid hyperplasia.[1] In a study surveying ENT physicians on the signs likely to be used to diagnose LPR, laryngeal erythema and edema were the most common.[9,10] However, reports from a study indicate that several signs of posterior laryngitis that have been considered to be signs of LPR are present in a high percentage of asymptomatic healthy volunteers raising question on their diagnostic specificity.[3]

Based on a study of pH-confirmed LPR patients, some have advocated the use of the Reflux Symptom Index (RSI). This is a self-administered tool that helps clinicians assess the clinical severity of LPR symptoms at diagnosis and then after treatment. Patients rate 9 symptoms such as throat clearing, hoarseness, and difficulty swallowing on a scale from 0 to 5. The RSI is significantly higher in untreated LPR patients than in controls (21.2 vs 11.6, p <.001). Any score greater than 13 is considered abnormal.[11] However, this index is seldom used by the general ENT practitioners.[9]

DIAGNOSIS

The diagnosis of LPR is most commonly suspected on the basis of combination of chronic throat symptoms and laryngeal findings. However, given lack of specificity of symptoms and signs for GERD many patients initially diagnosed with LPR do not respond to treatment for GERD and will need evaluation for other potential causes. Other potential causes for patient's persistent symptoms and laryngeal signs may include tobacco, alcohol, allergies, vocal trauma, vocal fold overuse or abuse, infections, or postnasal discharge.

The two most commonly used diagnostic tools in LPR include laryngoscopy and pH monitoring. There are numerous signs on laryngoscopy that are attributed to reflux disease: edema and erythema of the larynx, granuloma, contact ulcers, polyps, subglottic stenosis, tumors, or cobblestoning of posterior pharynx (hyperemia and lymphoid hyperplasia).[12] However, a survey of 2,000 ENT physicians revealed that the two signs most likely to be used to diagnose laryngitis associated with reflux were erythema and edema of the larynx.[9] These signs are highly nonspecific and many healthy adults have laryngeal changes without any throat symptoms.[3] Additionally, "abnormal" laryngeal signs are more likely to be suspected with flexible than with rigid laryngoscopes, suggesting that flexible laryngoscopy is more sensitive but less specific in identifying laryngeal tissue irritation.[13] Finally, a recent study evaluated the prevalence of laryngeal signs in GERD versus non-GERD controls and found that there was no difference among most laryngeal signs between the groups, suggesting lack of diagnostic specificity of laryngeal signs for GERD.[14] Therefore, it appears that laryngeal signs are poorly specific for LPR, which can explain why patients initially diagnosed with reflux-related laryngitis often do not respond to appropriate treatment.[15] More specific signs need to be identified to increase the rate of correct diagnoses of LPR. In one study, vocal fold lesions were suggested to represent more specific signs for LPR with 91% specificity and 88% response to PPI therapy.[16]

In addition to the nonspecificity of the currently employed signs in LPR, an additional problem is the inter- and intraobserver variability of laryngoscopic exam. One study which recorded ENT physician's independent ratings of laryngeal images of 120 patients revealed poor inter- and intrarater reliability.[17] Additionally, there is poor correlation between symptoms and laryngoscopic findings. This was evidenced in a recent study where patients with LPR symptoms who were refractory to aggressive PPI therapy underwent a Nissen fundoplication. One year postfundoplication, laryngeal symptoms improved in only 10% of patients, whereas signs improved in 80%.[18]

The Reflux Finding Score (RFS)[19] is a laryngoscopic evaluation tool developed to improve the reliability between ENT physicians. It consists of an 8-item, semiobjective, clinical severity scale for ENT physicians to use when evaluating findings at laryngoscopy. Each of the 8 items are ranked from either 0 to 2 or 0 to 4 with a Reflux Finding Score of 7 or more indicating a 95% chance that the patient indeed does have LPR. Initial studies found good inter- and intraobserver reproducibility for this tool in assessment and follow-up of LPR patients.[19] However, similar to RSI, RFS is seldom used in clinical or academic practice as it is not user friendly and somewhat cumbersome to remember. Finally, the clinical relevance of the RFS is in question. The reliability of this score has recently been questioned.[20,21]

When the diagnosis is in question, ambulatory 24-hour double-probe monitoring (simultaneous esophageal and pharyngeal monitoring) is believed by some to be useful in the diagnosis in LPR. Compared with physical exam findings, dual pH-probe monitoring does have superior sensitivity and specificity.[7] However, there is much variability in testing methods and lack of agreement on what pH value is considered abnormal. Additionally, one study determined that it was a poor predictor of the severity of patients' symptoms and signs.[22] A more recent meta-analysis involving 16 studies and 793 subjects who underwent 24-hour pH monitoring (264 controls, 529 LPR patients) found that the number of positive pharyngeal reflux events for normal subjects and for subjects with LPR differed significantly. There was also a significant difference in acid exposure times between these two groups. The conclusion from this study was that the "upper probe gives accurate and consistent information in normal subjects and patients with LPR" and that the acid exposure time and number of reflux events are most important in distinguishing normal subjects from patients with LPR.[23]

However, there are numerous problems with using pH data to diagnose LPR. First, several studies have shown that proximal esophageal and hypopharyngeal acid exposure occurs in normal subjects as well (from 7 to 17%).[24-26] Second, there are no universally accepted diagnostic criteria for hypopharyngeal pH monitoring (normal pH limits, number of events, and probe placement). Finally, proximal and hypopharyngeal probes have poor sensitivity in detecting reflux of gastric acid, 50% and 40%, respectively.[27,28]

The most recent pH system is the Restech Dx-pH Measurement System™ which is a new highly sensitive and minimally invasive device for detection of acid reflux in the posterior oropharynx. It uses a nasopharyngeal catheter able to measure pH in either liquid or aerosolized droplets. The probe is a 1.5-mm diameter oropharyngeal catheter with wireless digital ZigBee™ transmitter on the shirt collar. The catheter employs a 3.2-mm teardrop tip to aid in insertion and to ensure that the sensor is positioned in the airway. The tip has a colored Light-emitting diode (LED), for oral visualization. The sensing element consists of a circular 1-mm antimony surface and a reference electrode separated by a 0.05-mm polymer insulator. Moisture from exhaled air condenses on the sensor surface creating a fluid layer, which bridges the gap between the antimony and reference sensor elements. The sensor records pH values twice every second (2 Hz) and it features a hydration monitor to eliminate data if the tip dries out. Special circuitry monitors each individual reading to ensure sufficient sensor hydration. This circuitry prevents the inclusion of dry out-related "pseudoreflux" events in the data. The potential clinical utility of this device is in patients with extraesophageal reflux disease. Clinical data are needed to assess future role for this new device.

Given poor specificity of laryngoscopic exam and poor sensitivity of pH monitoring, the most accepted method employed in clinical practice to suggest the diagnosis of LPR is an empiric trial of a proton-pump inhibitor. Other diagnostic tests, such as barium esophagraphy or esophagoscopy, are far less sensitive for LPR than laryngoscopy or pH monitoring and thus offer little in the diagnosis and management of this group of patients.

The role of nonacid reflux in those who remain symptomatic on PPI therapy is recently gaining some popularity.[29-32] Employing the newly developed combined impedance and pH monitoring may shed light on this possible mechanism of disease. Combining these two techniques allows for the detection of all reflux events and distinction to be made between acid, weakly acidic, and weakly alkaline reflux.[30] Impedance works by measuring changes in resistance to alternating current between a series of metal electrodes produced by gas, liquid, or bolus. Metal rings are placed on a catheter to determine the impedance (increased by gas and decreased by liquid). Measuring impedance at multiple sites (multichannel) allows for determination of the direction of the esophageal bolus (antegrade vs retrograde).

A recent multicenter trial, which used impedance-pH-metry in healthy adults, has provided normal values that can be used in clinical and research settings for comparison with reflux patients.[33] Recent data from a single center[34] and multicenter[31] studies in a group of patients with heartburn and regurgitation as well as those with extraesophageal symptoms suggested that 10% to 40% of patients on BID PPI therapy may have continued nonacid reflux. However, the causal association between these reflux events and patients' continued reflux symptoms are difficult to establish. Preliminary outcomes data on response of this group of patients to surgical fundoplication[32] are encouraging and await validation by large-scale multicenter controlled trials.

TREATMENT

Initial treatment of LPR patients should include education about the disorder and recommendations regarding diet and behavioral changes that may play a role in the pathophysiology. Ideally, foods and beverages containing caffeine, alcohol, chocolate, and peppermints that are thought to weaken the esophageal sphincters and possibly increase acid secretion, should be eliminated. Carbonated beverages, with or without caffeine, are thought to worsen reflux as it often prompts belching, allowing gastric contents to bypass the protective esophageal sphincters. Additionally, acidic foods (pH below 4.6) should be limited. This includes citrus fruits, tomatoes, and red wines. Other lifestyle modifications that may improve LPR symptoms, as well as other symptoms of extraesophageal reflux, include smoking cessation and weight loss. A study by Steward et al[35] revealed that lifestyle modification for 2 months, with or without PPI therapy, significantly improved chronic laryngitis symptoms.

Drug therapy usually consists of acid suppression with proton-pump inhibitors (PPI's). As both laryngoscopy and pH monitoring are not 100% accurate in diagnosis, empiric therapy with a PPI is warranted, especially as it may aid in diagnosis. To date, studies examining the efficacy of PPI therapy in LPR patients have produced a broad range of responses. This is most likely due to selection biases and the true prevalence of reflux-induced laryngeal disease. Most uncontrolled studies suggest near 70% response rate with PPIs.[36] However, nearly all controlled studies disappointingly do not suggest a major benefit of PPIs over placebo. An earlier controlled trial involving treatment with lanoprazole 30 mg twice daily for 3 months in 22 patients with idiopathic chronic laryngitis revealed that 50% of the treatment group had a complete response versus 10% in the control group.[37] However, another study using the same medicine regimen, found no difference in response rates in patients with posterior pharyngolaryngitis.[38] The most recent large scale multicenter study of 145 patients suspected of having LPR did not show a benefit in those treated for 4 months with esomeprazole 40 mg BID compared to placebo.[39] Although, a disappointing result, once again this study highlights the difficulty in certainty of the LPR diagnosis in most patients. Similarly, Wo et al[40] found no difference between pantoprazole

40 mg once daily versus placebo in patients newly diagnosed with LPR. Finally, meta-analysis of the 8 controlled studies in LPR (Fig 3-1) showed that PPI therapy may offer a modest, but nonsignificant, clinical benefit over placebo in suspected LPR patients.[41]

Given the negative findings of controlled trials, currently uncontrolled studies are the basis for the treatment recommendations in patients with LPR. Two studies which both examined use of omeprazole 40 mg (initially once-daily dosing which was changed to twice-daily dosing in nonresponders) reported response rates of 67% and 92%.[42,43] All of the above studies were limited by small numbers and short duration. The most recent study involving 85 subjects determined that twice-daily PPI therapy was more efficacious than once-daily therapy and that extending therapy to 4 months from 2 months resulted in more responses.[44] Overall, the general consensus supports the use of twice-daily PPI therapy for 2 to 3 months. Unlike GERD, the variable efficacy of PPI therapy for LPR suggest the multifactorial nature of the disease process.

The role of combination therapy of PPIs with histamine-2 receptor antagonists (H2RA) was initially raised by Peghini et al[45] in 1998 when it was determined that three-fourths of patients experienced a return of pH <4 for greater than 1 hour within 12 hours of their evening PPI dose. A follow-up study by Peghini et al[46] examined whether a bedtime histamine-2

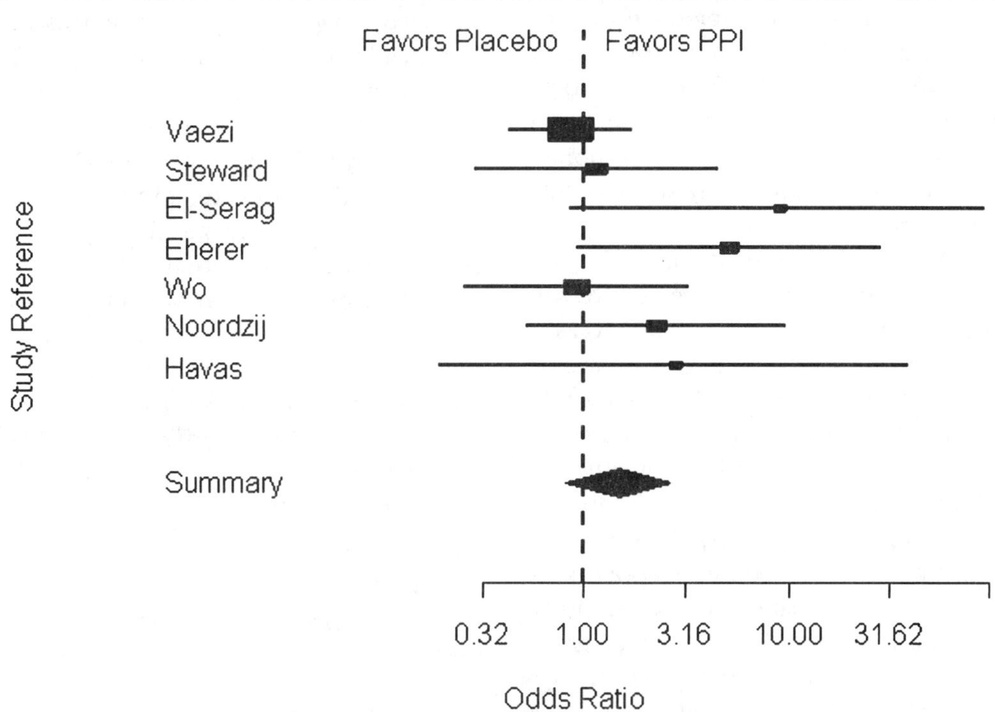

Fig 3–1. Forest plot depicting the odds ratio and 95% confidence intervals for each placebo-controlled PPI treatment trials for LPR.

receptor antagonist (H2RA, ranitidine) or a bedtime PPI dose would be beneficial in patients on BID dosing of a PPI with nocturnal acid breakthrough (NAB). It was determined that a bedtime ranitidine rather than a 3rd dose of a PPI at bedtime was more effective on NAB. However, two later studies examining the role of H2RA's for NAB concluded that H2RA's provide no additional benefit over PPI therapy alone.[47,48] The current recommendations do not suggest the use of nocturnal H2RA in addition to PPIs in patients suspected of LPR. To achieve best results, PPIs should be taken on an empty stomach, about 30 minutes before a meal.

Treatment with a PPI usually will result in improving patient symptoms within 1 month of therapy[49] but laryngeal signs may take up to 6 months to resolve.[11] Patients who do not improve after 1 to 2 months of therapy most likely do not have GERD as the cause of their laryngeal signs and throat symptoms. However, they may need to be tested for nonacid reflux using the combined impedance/pH monitoring while on BID PPI therapy.

The role of surgical fundoplication in those poorly responsive to BID PPI therapy is still somewhat controversial. A recent study[18] evaluated 12-month symptomatic response of 10 patients who despite lack of response to PPI therapy underwent fundoplication compared to 12 PPI unresponsive patients who continued on their therapy. They showed that only 10% of patients responded to surgical fundoplication and this response rate was not any different from the group who continued on their PPI therapy (7%). Thus, they suggested that surgical fundoplication does not reliably relieve symptoms in LPR patients who were unresponsive to medical management. However, the role of surgical intervention in the subgroup of PPI unresponsive patients who have abnormal nonacid reflux detected by impedance monitoring suggests that these patients can be successfully treated by laparoscopic Nissen fundoplication.[32] A large scale randomized, controlled outcome study is currently underway to assess the efficacy of surgical fundoplication in symptomatic patients on therapy who have abnormal nonacid reflux on impedance monitoring.

CONCLUSIONS

Common clinical manifestations of LPR include dysphonia, cough, globus pharyngeus, throat clearing, and dysphagia. Unless they report warning symptoms, this group of patients should be treated empirically consisting of lifestyle modification as well as twice-daily PPI therapy for 1 to 2 months. Patients whose symptoms resolve should have tapering of the medication dose to minimum acid suppression that keeps them in the asymptomatic state. Patients who show minimal or no sign of improvement after adequate trial of PPIs, will require physiologic assessment to ensure adequate acid and nonacid reflux as the contributing factors. Etiologies other than reflux should be investigated in most patients unresponsive to PPIs.

REFERENCES

1. Vaezi MF, Hicks DM, Abelson TI, Richter JE. Laryngeal signs and symptoms and gastroesophageal reflux disease: a critical

assessment of cause and effect association. *Clin Gastroenterol Hepatol.* 2003; 1:333-344.

2. Ford CN. Evaluation and management of laryngopharyngeal reflux. *JAMA.* 2005; 294:1534-1540.
3. Hicks DM, Ours TM, Abelson TI, Vaezi MF, Richter JE. The prevalence of hypopharynx findings associated with gastroesophageal reflux in normal volunteers. *J Voice.* 2002;16:564-579.
4. Hanson DG, Jiang JJ. Diagnosis and management of chronic laryngitis associated with reflux. *Am J Med.* 2000;108: 112S-119S.
5. Loughlin CJ, Koufman JA, Averill DB, et al. Acid-induced laryngospasm in a canine model. *Laryngoscope.* 1996;106: 1506-1509.
6. Adhami T, Goldblum JR, Richter JE, Vaezi MF. The role of gastric and duodenal agents in laryngeal injury: an experimental canine model. *Am J Gastroenterol.* 2004;99:2098-2106.
7. Koufman JA. The otolaryngologic manifestations of gastroesophageal reflux disease (GERD): a clinical investigation of 225 patients using ambulatory 24-hour pH monitoring and an experimental investigation of the role of acid and pepsin in the development of laryngeal injury. *Laryngoscope.* 1991;101:1-78.
8. Koufman JA, Amin MR, Panetti M. Prevalence of reflux in 113 consecutive patients with laryngeal and voice disorders. *Otolaryngol Head Neck Surg.* 2000; 123:385-388.
9. Ahmed TF, Khandwala F, Abelson TI, et al. Chronic laryngitis associated with gastroesophageal reflux: prospective assessment of differences in practice patterns between gastroenterologists and ENT physicians. *Am J Gastroenterol.* 2006; 101:470-478.
10. Book DT, Rhee JS, Toohill RJ, Smith TL. Perspectives in laryngopharyngeal reflux: an international survey. *Laryngoscope.* 2002;112:1399-1406.
11. Belafsky PC, Postma GN, Koufman JA. Validity and reliability of the reflux symptom index (RSI). *J Voice.* 2002;16: 274-277.
12. Al-Sabbagh G, Wo JM. Supraesophageal manifestations of gastroesophageal reflux disease. *Semin Gastrointest Dis.* 1999; 10:113-119.
13. Milstein CF, Charbel S, Hicks DM, Abelson TI, Richter JE, Vaezi MF. Prevalence of laryngeal irritation signs associated with reflux in asymptomatic volunteers: impact of endoscopic technique (rigid vs flexible laryngoscope. *Laryngoscope.* 2005;115:2256-2261.
14. Vavricka SR, Storkc CA, Wildi SM, et al. Limited diagnostic value of laryngopharyngeal lesions in patients with gastroesophageal reflux during routine upper gastrointestinal endoscopy. *Am J Gastroenterol.* 2007;102:716-722.
15. Vaezi MF. Are there specific laryngeal signs for GERD? *Am J Gastroenterol.* 2007;102:723-724.
16. Park W, Hicks DM, Khandwala F, et al. Laryngopharyngeal reflux: prospective cohort study evaluating optimal dose of proton-pump inhibitor therapy and pretherapy predictors of response. *Laryngoscope.* 2005;115:1230-1238.
17. Branski RC, Bhattacharyya N, Shapiro J. The reliability of the assessment of endoscopic laryngeal findings associated with laryngopharyngeal reflux disease. *Laryngoscope.* 2002;112:1019-1024.
18. Swoger J, Ponsky J, Hicks DM, et al. Surgical fundoplication in laryngopharyngeal reflux unresponsive to aggressive acid suppression: a controlled study. *Clin Gastroenterol Hepatol.* 2006;4:433-441.
19. Belafsky PC, Postma GN, Koufman JA. The validity and reliability of the reflux finding score (RFS). *Laryngoscope.* 2001; 111:1313-1317.
20. Branski RC, Bhattacharyya N, Shaprio J. Thee reliability of the assessment of endoscopic laryngeal findings associated with laryngopharyngeal reflux disease. *Laryngoscope.* 2002;112:1019-1024.

21. Kelchner LN, Horne J, Lee L, et al. Reliability of speech-language pathologist and otolaryngologist ratings of laryngeal signs of reflux in an asymptomatic population using the reflux finding score. *J Voice.* 2007;21:92–100.
22. Noordzij JP, Khidr A, Desper E, Meek RB, Reibel JF, Levine PA. Correlation of pH probe-measured laryngopharyngeal reflux with symptoms and signs of reflux laryngitis. *Laryngoscope.* 2002;112:2192–2195.
23. Merati AL, Lim HJ, Ulualp SO, Toohill RJ. Meta-analysis of upper probe measurements in normal subjects and patients with laryngopharyngeal reflux. *Ann Otol Rhinol Laryngol.* 2005;114:177–182.
24. Jacob P, Kahrilas PJ, Herzon G. Proximal esophageal pH-metry in patients with "reflux laryngitis." *Gastroenterology.* 1991;100:305–310.
25. Shaker R, Milbrath M, Ren J, et al. Esophagopharyngeal distribution of refluxed gastric acid in patients with reflux laryngitis. *Gastroenterology.* 1995;109:1575–1582.
26. Eubanks TR, Omelanczuk PE, Maronian N, Hillel A, Pope CE 2nd, Pellegrini CA. Pharyngeal pH monitoring in 222 patients with suspected laryngeal reflux. *J Gastrointest Surg.* 2001;5:183–190.
27. Vaezi MF, Schroeder PL, Richter JE. Reproducibility of proximal probe pH parameters in 24-hour ambulatory esophageal pH monitoring. *Am J Gastroenterol.* 1997;92:825–829.
28. Kawamura O, Aslam M, Rittmann T, Hofmann C, Shaker R. Physical and pH properties of gastroesophagopharyngeal refluxate: a 24-hour simultaneous ambulatory impedance and pH monitoring study. *Am J Gastroenterol.* 2004;99(6):1020–1022.
29. Vaezi MF. Reflux-induced laryngitis. *Curr Treat Options Gastroenterol.* 2006;9:69–74.
30. Sifrim D, Blondeau K. Technology insight: the role of impedance testing for esophageal disorders. *Nat Clin Pract Gastroenterol Hepatol.* 2006;3:210–219.
31. Mainie I, Tutuian R, Shay S, et al. Acid and non-acid reflux in patients with persistent symptoms despite acid suppressive therapy: a multicentre study using combined ambulatory impedance-pH monitoring. *Gut.* 2006;55:1398–1402.
32. Mainie I, Tutuian R, Agrawal A, Adams D, Castell DO. Combined multichannel intraluminal impedance-pH monitoring to select patients with persistent gastro-oesophageal reflux for laparoscopic Nissen fundoplication. *Br J Surg.* 2006;93:1483–1487.
33. Shay S, Tutuian R, Sifrim D, et al. Twenty-four hour ambulatory simultaneous impedance and pH monitoring: a multicenter report of normal values from 60 healthy volunteers. *Am J Gastroenterol.* 2004;99:1037–1043.
34. Vaezi MF, Hicks DM, Ours TM, Richter JE. ENT manifestation of GERD: a large prospective study assessing treatment outcome and predictors of response. *Gastroenterology.* 2001;120:A636.
35. Steward DL, Wilson KM, Kelly DH, et al. Proton pump inhibitor therapy for chronic laryngo-pharyngitis: a randomized placebo-control trial. *Otolaryngol Head Neck Surg.* 2004;131:342–350.
36. Vaezi MF. Extraesophageal manifestations of gastroesophageal reflux disease. *Clin Cornerstone.* 2003;5:32–38.
37. El-Serag HB, Lee P, Buchner A, Inadomi JM, Gavin M, McCarthy DM. Lansoprazole treatment of patients with chronic idiopathic laryngitis: a placebo-controlled trial. *Am J Gastroenterol.* 200;96:979–983.
38. Havas T, Huang S, Levy M, et al. Posterior pharyngolaryngitis: double blind randomized placebo controlled trial of proton pump inhibitor therapy. *Aust J Otolaryngol.* 1999;3:243–246.
39. Vaezi MF, Richter JE, Stasney CR, et al. Treatment of chronic posterior laryngitis with esomeprazole. *Laryngoscope.* 2006;116:254–260.
40. Wo JM, Koopman J, Harrell SP, Parker K, Winstead W, Lentsch E. Double blind,

placebo controlled trial with single dose pantoprazole for laryngopharyngeal reflux. *Am J Gastroenterol.* 2006;101: 1972-1978.

41. Qadeer MA, Phillips CO, Lopez AR, et al. Proton pump inhibitor therapy for suspected GERD-related chronic laryngitis: a meta-analysis of randomized controlled trials. *Am J Gastroenterol.* 2006;101: 2646-2654.
42. Kamel PL, Hanson D, Kahrilas PJ. Omeprazole for the treatment of posterior laryngitis. *Am J Med.* 1994;96:321-326.
43. Wo JM, Grist WJ, Gussack G, Delgaudio JM, Waring JP. Empiric trial of high-dose omeprazole in patients with posterior laryngitis: a prospective study. *Am J Gastroenterol.* 1997;92:2160-2165.
44. Park W, Hicks DM, Khandwala F, et al. Laryngopharyngeal reflux: prospective cohort study evaluating optimal dose of proton-pump inhibitor therapy and pretherapy predictors of response. *Laryngoscope.* 2005;115:1230-1238.
45. Peghini PL, Katz PO, Bracy NA, Castell DO. Nocturnal recovery of gastric acid secretion with twice-daily dosing of proton pump inhibitors. *Am J Gastroenterol.* 1998;93:763-767.
46. Peghini PL, Katz PO, Castell DO. Ranitidine controls nocturnal gastric acid breakthrough on omeprazole: a controlled study in normal subjects. *Gastroenterology.* 1998;115:1335-1339.
47. Fackler WK, Ours TM, Vaezi MF, Richter JE. Long-term effect of H2RA therapy on nocturnal gastric acid breakthrough. *Gastroenterology.* 2002;122:625-632.
48. Ours TM, Fackler WK, Richter JE, Vaezi MF. Nocturnal acid breakthrough: clinical significance and correlation with esophageal acid exposure. *Am J Gastroenterol.* 2003;98:545-550.
49. Vaezi MF, Lopez R, Hicks D, Abelson T, Milstein C. What is the optimal initial therapy duration for patients with suspected GERD-related laryngitis? *Gastroenterology.* 2005;128:M1769.

4

Laryngopharyngeal Reflux from the Otolaryngologist's Perspective

Paul M. Weinberger and Gregory N. Postma

INTRODUCTION

Laryngopharyngeal reflux (LPR) continues to be a controversial disease process, as evident by a continued lack of definitive diagnostic criteria. Nevertheless, it is also very real, and impacts hundreds of thousands of patients annually. Some authors estimate as many as 30% of Americans may suffer from some degree of LPR.[1] The prevalence of reflux disease is markedly higher in patients with voice disorders, as high as 50%.[2] While our understanding of LPR continues to evolve, one fact is consistently clear—LPR is a related yet distinct disorder from classic gastro-esophageal reflux disease (GERD).[3-7] It is clearly evident that no single symptom, or laryngeal finding, can be used as a stand-alone diagnostic feature; rather, the gestalt of the severity of the patient's symptoms, laryngoscopic findings, and diagnostic testing, should be taken into consideration to reach a diagnosis. In this chapter we present LPR as viewed from the otolaryngologist's perspective with an emphasis on current best-practice guidelines for diagnosing LPR using a combination of symptoms and laryngoscopic findings.

RELEVANT PATHOPHYSIOLOGY

Numerous physiologic barriers protect the upper aerodigestive tract, including the larynx, from reflux-mediated injury. The lower esophageal sphincter and upper esophageal sphincter function as physiologic valves preventing retrograde passage of gastric contents. Additionally, normal esophageal peristalsis acts to clear any refluxed acid from the esophagus by propelling it distally back into the stomach and the acidic residue is neutralized by dilution and salivary bicarbonate (esophageal acid clearance).[8] Any refluxate that bypasses these physical protective mechanisms must then overcome mucosal resistance to produce injury and subsequent clinical consequences.[4,8] However, unlike the esophagus' relatively resistant stratified squamous epithelium, the posterior laryngeal mucosa is composed of more delicate ciliated respiratory epithelium. Although the true vocal folds are covered by stratified squamous epithelium, the remainder of the laryngeal mucosa lacks at a molecular level some of the cellular defenses present in esophageal mucosa.[8,9] This difference in molecular protective barriers in part may account for the lack of traditional GERD symptoms in many LPR patients. Even small amounts of refluxate may damage the delicate laryngeal mucosa; up to 50 acid exposure events per day in the esophagus still fall within the normal physiologic range; whereas, it has been proposed that one or two episodes of acid exposure to the laryngeal mucosa in 24 hours may be abnormal.[6] Several authors have demonstrated decreased expression of E-cadherin (a cell adhesion constituent) and carbonic anhydrase (a key enzyme in acid-base homeostasis) in the laryngeal mucosa of LPR patients.[10-12] Carbonic anhydrase catalyzes the conversion of carbon dioxide to bicarbonate; this may serve as a protective mechanism to prevent laryngeal damage from acidic refluxate.[12]

In addition to acid exposure causing direct laryngeal mucosal damage, it is becoming clear that LPR has a multifactorial etiology. In a study of symptomatic LPR patients on BID acid suppressive therapy, 99% had normal esophageal pH monitoring.[13] Thus, the PPI acid suppression therapy was working, but patients continued to experience LPR symptoms. It has been proposed that nonacid reflux may play a significant role in LPR.[14-16] As early as 1978, Pellegrini[17] first drew attention to alkaline reflux events. Later, Galli et al[18] proposed biliary reflux as possible contributor to LPR. In support of this, Sasaki et al[14] found that exposure of laryngeal mucosa to bile salts resulted in a profound inflammatory response in a rat model. Similarly, nonacidic bolus presence in the esophagus has been found to produce LPR-like symptoms temporarily.[16] In healthy controls, acidic reflux events to the proximal esophagus are not rare events (9 events per 24 hours) whereas nonacid reflux is virtually nonexistent.[20]

This contrasts sharply with findings in patients with LPR. Mainie et al[20] found that of 168 patients with LPR or GERD symptoms recalcitrant to PPI therapy, acid reflux events were rare (median of 1 event per 24 hours) and nonacid reflux events were common (20 events per 24 hours). Of particular interest, of 59 patients in this study with only LPR-specific symptoms (hoarseness, globus, subjectively increased mucus awareness),[12] 20% had nonacid reflux events that coincided timewise with their symptoms and none of these patients had acid reflux events coinciding with their symptoms.[20]

LPR-ASSOCIATED DISORDERS IN THE HEAD AND NECK

Historically, several authors have demonstrated an epidemiologic association between LPR and upper aerodigestive tract carcinoma[21-24] (reviewed in ref. 25). More recently, a large case-control study by Vaezi et al[26] found that smoking and GERD were independent risk factors for the development of laryngeal cancer. Although current evidence for this remains correlative, recent studies illuminating the link between chronic inflammation and cancer development lend plausibility to a possible etiologic link.[27-29] According to current theories, chronic inflammatory states (characterized by presence of macrophages, neutrophils, and mast cells) contribute to cancer development by multiple mechanisms. The first involves local growth factor and angiogenesis-promoting factor production. These secreted factors induce epithelial proliferation, and the resultant rapid cellular turnover can predispose to dysplastic progression. Secondly, free-radical production and other oxidative stressors from innate immune cells can result in DNA damage and progression to a malignant phenotype.

Laryngopharyngeal reflux has also been implicated in a host of other disorders of the head and neck, including obstructive sleep apnea (OSA),[30-36] chronic rhinosinusitis (CRS),[37-43] and subglottic stenosis.[44-49] The relationship of OSA with reflux (both GERD and LPR) deserves specific mention. Several studies have demonstrated a high degree of correlation between presence of OSA and either GERD[31,50] or LPR.[35] Both diseases share risk factors including obesity; it is intuitive that such commonality might explain the linkage. However, there is also evidence that some causality independent of the common risk factors may be at work. In a large study that included 204 patients with both OSA and GERD, Green et al[30] found that treatment of OSA (with CPAP) resulted in marked improvement of nighttime GERD events. This raises the possibility that obstructive events characteristic of untreated OSA may predispose to GERD. Intriguingly, the corollary also may be true. In a prospective clinical trial involving OSA patients with concomitant LPR, Friedman et al[51] recently demonstrated improvement in several clinical parameters associated with OSA following high-dose PPI therapy. These improvements were noted only for patients who responded to PPI therapy as measured by post-treatment 24-hour pH probe. Possible mechanisms for these relationships remain purely speculative at this time and further research is clearly indicated.

Patient Presentation and History

The typical presenting symptoms for a patient with LPR are quite different from classic GERD symptoms. The vast majority of GERD patients report heartburn (83%) whereas only 20% of LPR patients report this symptom.[4] Similarly, 87% of patients with LPR report frequent throat clearing compared to only 3% of GERD patients.[52] Thus, the symptom set for LPR is separate from GERD symptoms. Other complaints common among LPR patients include cough, globus sensation, hoarseness or dysphonia, dysphagia, and excessive mucus production.[4,52-56] A summary of frequent LPR symptoms is presented in Table 4-1.

As can be seen from this list, individually many of the symptoms associated with LPR are also quite common in presumably normal patients. Additionally, these symptoms can be caused by a multitude of processes in addition to or instead of LPR-related damage.[53,54] In order to help elucidate which symptoms or combination of symptoms are most predictive of true LPR, several authors have devised symptom indexes. The most widely accepted of these is the Reflux Symptom Index, or RSI (Table 4–2).[56] This is a well-validated test in the form of a nine-item self-administered questionnaire.[57] RSI scores range from 0 (no symptoms) to a maximum of 45. The RSI has been extensively validated for use in assessing the relative severity of LPR symptoms both at initial presentation and following treatment.[56] Belafsky et al[56] demonstrated that the pretreatment RSI in LPR patients was 21.2 as compared to 11.6 in healthy controls. An RSI of greater than 13 was derived as an abnormal value indicative of a high likelihood of LPR.

Table 4–1. Common Symptoms Associated with LPR

Symptoms Frequently Associated with LPR	Reference
Globus sensation	(52, 55, 56)
Frequent throat clearing	(52, 55, 56)
Cough	(55, 56)
Hoarseness	(52, 54–56)
Throat pain	(54)
Sensation of excessive mucus	(56)

Physical Findings (Transnasal Laryngoscopy)

Traditionally understood physical exam findings (ie, that which the clinician can observe or elicit directly by examination, auscultation, palpation and percussion) are not useful in the diagnosis of LPR. Rather, otolaryngologists rely on visualization of the affected organs, the pharynx and larynx, usually by flexible transnasal laryngoscopy. Tremendous technologic advancements in the last

Table 4–2. Reflux Symptom Index, or RSI

Within the last MONTH, how did the following problem affect you?	0 = no problem 5 = severe problem
1. Hoarseness or a problem with your voice	0 1 2 3 4 5
2. Clearing your throat	0 1 2 3 4 5
3. Excess throat mucus or postnasal drip	0 1 2 3 4 5
4. Difficulty swallowing food, liquids, or pills	0 1 2 3 4 5
5. Coughing after you ate or after lying down	0 1 2 3 4 5
6. Breathing difficulties or choking episodes	0 1 2 3 4 5
7. Troublesome or annoying cough	0 1 2 3 4 5
8. Sensations of something sticking in your throat or a lump in your throat	0 1 2 3 4 5
9. Heartburn, chest pain, indigestion, or stomach acid coming up	0 1 2 3 4 5

Patients are asked to rate on a scale of 0 to 5 how each problem has affected them within the last month.
From: Belafsky et al. *J Voice.* 2002;16(2):274–277. Used with permission.

two decades have resulted in a progression from mirror-based indirect laryngoscopy to rigid transoral laryngoscopy to flexible fiberoptic-based laryngoscopy. With the advent of high-resolution distal-chip laryngoscopes, unprecedented visualization of the larynx and pharynx are now available in many laryngology practices. These advances notwithstanding, many otolaryngologists still rely primarily on symptoms when diagnosing LPR, with laryngoscopic findings providing supporting evidence.[54]

The importance of a laryngeal examination in evaluating patients with suspected LPR cannot be overstressed. Many of the symptoms found in LPR are also present in other disorders. Hoarseness in particular deserves specific mention. Any pathophysiologic process that alters the way air flows over the vocal folds can produce hoarseness. This list includes LPR, vocal fold paresis, polyps, postviral inflammatory reaction, allergy, vocal abuse, dysplasia, and cancer.[54] Thus, persistent or progressive hoarseness lasting longer than 2 weeks necessitates a laryngeal examination.

Common laryngoscopic findings consistent with LPR are posterior laryngeal hypertrophy[58] and laryngeal edema and erythema,[4,53–55,59] especially of the medial aspect of the arytenoids and the posterior true vocal folds.[60,61] Other common findings include presence of cobblestoning, a posterior commisure bar, vocal fold granuloma, and laryngeal pseudosulcus (ie, infraglottic edema).[54,61,62] Laryngeal pseudosulcus (Color Plate 3A) is caused by diffuse infraglottic edema of the true vocal folds extending from the anterior commisure to the posterior larynx, creating what appears to be a linear indentation of the medial edge of the vocal fold.[4,62] This can be confused with sulcus vocalis (Color Plate 3B), in which fibrosis and tissue loss of the lamina propria leads to a true indentation that stops at the vocal process. In contrast, in pseudosulcus the concavity is due to diffuse edema in the surrounding tissues and extends the length of the entire vocal fold. Although some authors have reported laryngeal pseudosulcus in up to 90% of patients with LPR,[62] subsequent studies have shown slightly lower prevalence in LPR patients. Belafsky et al[63] demonstrated presence of laryngeal pseudosulcus to be highly suggestive of, but not pathognomonic for, LPR with a sensitivity of 70% and specificity of 77%. A summary of common LPR-related findings is presented in Table 4–3 and Color Plate 4.

As is the case with LPR-related symptoms, many of the laryngoscopic findings above can be demonstrated in healthy presumably normal patients. Several investigators have demonstrated the presence of at least one LPR-related laryngoscopic finding in 83 to 93% of healthy, nonsmoking normal volunteers.[66,67] These laryngoscopic findings therefore are not *individually* diagnostic for LPR but rather represent phenotypic expressions of a final common pathway for laryngeal irritation, injury, and inflammatory response.

Given the lack of an individually pathognomonic laryngoscopic finding, the Wake Forest group found that using a combination of LPR-related findings results in improved accuracy in diagnosis LPR compared to isolated findings alone. The resulting clinical instrument (Table 4–4), the Reflux Finding Score (RFS), has been validated and is widely used.[57,58] This instrument is a composite of 8 common LPR-related laryngoscopic findings, with possible scores ranging from 0 (no LPR-related findings) to 26 (the worst possible

Table 4–3. Laryngoscopic Findings Associated with LPR

Findings Predictive for LPR	Reference
Diffuse laryngeal erythema or edema	(4, 53–55, 58–61)
Posterior laryngeal hypertrophy	(58)
Posterior commisure bar	(55)
Specific arytenoid and interarytenoid erythema or edema	(54, 58, 60)
Vocal fold granuloma	(54, 64)
Cobblestoning	(55)
Laryngeal pseudosulcus	(54, 58, 62, 63)
Ventricular obliteration	(58)
Thick endolaryngeal mucous	(58)
Nonspecific Findings Not Predictive for LPR	**Reference**
Pachydermia	(65)
Vocal fold nodules	(55)
Vocal fold polyps	(55)
Leuokoplakia	(55)

Table 4–4. Reflux Finding Score, or RFS

Laryngeal Finding	Points
Subglottic edema	Absent (0); Present (2)
Ventricular obliteration	Partial (2); Complete (4)
Erythema/hyperemia	Arytenoids only (2); Diffuse (4)
Vocal fold edema	Mild (1); Moderate (2); Severe (3); Polypoid (4)
Diffuse laryngeal edema	Mild (1); Moderate (2); Severe (3); Obstructing (4)
Posterior commisure hypertrophy	Mild (1); Moderate (2); Severe (3); Obstructing (4)
Granuloma/granulation tissue	Absent (0); Present (2)
Thick endolaryngeal mucus	Absent (0); Present (2)

From Belafsky PC, Postma GN, Koufman JA. The validity and reliability of the reflux finding score (RFS). *Laryngoscope.* 2001;111(8):1313–1317. Copyright 2001 by Lippincott-Williams and Wilkins.

score). A score on the RFS greater than 7 is accepted to be suggestive of LPR.[58] In addition to usefulness in diagnosing LPR, the RFS can be utilized to follow response to therapy over time.[54,68]

Diagnosis of LPR

It is important to emphasize that a diagnosis of LPR should not be made based on laryngeal findings alone. Indeed, most otolaryngologists make a diagnosis of LPR based on the combination of an appropriate set of presenting symptoms combined with response of these symptoms to empiric medical therapy.[15,54,55] Laryngoscopic findings, especially edema and erythema, can be used to support a diagnosis of LPR but should not be used as stand-alone diagnostic criteria. In general, an RSI greater than 13 is considered consistent with a diagnosis of LPR. Similarly, an RFS greater than 7 is associated with a high likelihood of extraesophageal reflux.

Once a diagnosis of LPR is arrived at, we recommend eventual endoscopic evaluation of the upper digestive tract via unsedated transnasal esophagoscopy (TNE) or conventional sedated esophagoscopy to evaluate for concurrent esophageal disease.[15] The authors recommend doing this after 4 to 6 weeks of antireflux therapy. Although the incidence of unsuspected esophageal abnormalities such as Barrett's esophagus is lower in LPR patients (20%) than in GERD patients (50%), identifying these patients is important as symptoms may be masked by empiric therapy.[69] An important subgroup of reflux patients requiring esophagoscopy are those with chronic cough. Reavis et al[21] have demonstrated that individuals with extraesophageal symptoms of reflux are more likely to have metaplastic changes of the esophagus than those with classic GERD symptoms.

Further studies such as pH monitoring, impedence studies, manometry, radiography, and mucosal biopsy can add useful information for the clinician but are less routinely used in the establishment of a diagnoses.[15] Although pH monitoring is of proven value for GERD, its role in diagnosing LPR remains undefined. Several authors have demonstrated poor predictive values for pH monitoring in LPR.[70-72] Although there is a strong statistical association of pharyngeal acid events with LPR, a significant portion (30–40%) of patients strongly suspected to have LPR lack demonstrable pharyngeal acid events by pH probe.[72] Similarly, Oelschlager et al[73] found that of 76 patients with suspected LPR, only 21 had both abnormal laryngeal findings (RFS >7) and pharyngeal acid events on pH probe. Compounding this problem, Shaker et al[74] demonstrated up to 20% of normal volunteers have pharyngeal acid events on pH monitoring.

Interpretation of pH-monitoring studies in LPR is further complicated by a lack of clearly defined normative values, and variability in anatomic location of the proximal probe. Placement of the proximal probe in the hypopharynx can allow intermittent drying of the pH probe resulting in false reports of acid events.[75] Conversely, placement of the proximal probe below the upper esophageal sphincter (UES) fails to capture acid events at the site of interest and may overestimate laryngeal acid events.[15] Current consensus opinion regarding proper placement for pH probes in evaluating LPR is to use manometry rather than visual placement,[76] with the hypopharyngeal probe just above the manometric UES, and the distal esophageal probe 5 cm above the manometric LES.[15] Even with proper probe placement, interpretation of the resulting study remains controversial. It appears that rather than strictly numerical counts of acid events, the acid exposure time percentage is most important in predicting patients with LPR.[77] Establishment of an abnormal pH threshold for the hypopharyngeal probe remains problematic. Current evidence, however, would suggest a pH cutpoint between 4 to 5 coincident with a distal probe acid event may be of most value.[77,78] In a meta-analysis of 16 double-probe pH studies, Merati et al[77] demonstrated a high degree of reliability in distinguishing normal controls from LPR patients when the above conditions are met. Specifically, upper pH probe placement 1 cm above the UES, and the use of acid-exposure times proved essential.

As mentioned earlier, nonacid reflux (NAR) or perhaps more accurately, weakly acidic reflux, may play a significant role in LPR.[14-16] This type of reflux is not detectable by conventional pH-monitoring studies, which detect presence of H+ ions. Relatively recent technology, such as multichannel intraluminal impedance (MII), allows discernment of presence of bolus within the esophagus.[79] When combined with pH monitoring (MII-pH), all reflux events can be detected and categorized as acidic reflux versus non-acidic reflux. Using MII-pH, Mainie et al[20] found up to 37% of symptomatic GERD patients had NAR events coincident with their symptoms.

One emerging technology holding future promise is the application of molecular biomarkers to the study of LPR. Biomarkers for LPR would be useful not only as an objective means of diagnosis, but also to monitor response to treatment. Possible biomarkers include epidermal growth factor,[80] laryngeal stress proteins,[81] E-cadherin,[10,11] pepsin, and carbonic anhydrase isoenzyme III (CAIII).[10,11,81,82] The combination of pepsin and CAIII appear particularly promising. In 2004 Johnston et al[82] demonstrated decreased expression of CAIII and increased pepsin deposition in laryngeal biopsies of LPR patients. Since then several authors have reported similar findings, and a pepsin assay has been proposed as a potential future diagnostic tool for LPR.[10,11,83]

Medical and Surgical Management

As stated earlier, LPR is a related yet distinct disease process from GERD. Thus, it stands to reason that treatment of LPR requires distinct management algorithms. Over-the-counter antacid medications (sodium bicarbonate, aluminum, and magnesium based), although efficacious for the relief of occasional GERD symptoms, lack efficacy in the treatement of LPR.[84] Likewise, there appears to be a poor response to histamine-2 receptor antagonists (H2RAs) in LPR patients.[15,54,85]

Lifestyle modifications play a role in the treatment of LPR, and patients should be counseled on abstaining from foods and beverages that cause symptoms for them. Avoidance of substances (alcohol, caffeine, nicotine) correlated with increased gastric reflux frequency or volume should be stressed.[86] Additional behavioral changes such as weight loss and elevation of the entire head of the bed can also be of benefit (Table 4-5). The importance of these nonpharmacologic interventions should be emphasized. Steward et al[87] demonstrated that short-term (2 month) improvements in LPR symptoms correlated strongly with patient lifestyle modification compliance, but not with use of PPI versus placebo. Longer term studies have demonstrated the usefulness of PPIs in the treatment of LPR,[88] but the contribution of lifestyle modifications cannot be ignored.

In contrast to H2RAs, proton-pump inhibitors (PPIs) directly target the H^+-K^+ ATPase enzyme responsible for secretion of H^+ ions and acid production. Their role in the treatment of GERD is well documented. Perhaps not surprisingly, given the likely multifactorial etiology of

Table 4–5. Dietary and Behavioral Modifications Recommended for LPR Patients

Behavioral Changes	Dietary Restrictions
Weight loss	Chocolate
Smoking cessation	Caffeine
Reduction in alcohol consumption	Fats
Elevate head of bed	Acidic foods (citrus fruits, tomato) products)
	Carbonated beverages
	Spicy foods
	Red wine
	Late-night meals

LPR, there is conflicting evidence in the literature regarding the efficacy of PPIs for the treatment of LPR. While several uncontrolled studies[89-91] and randomized controlled trials[88,92] have demonstrated efficacy of PPIs for the treatment of LPR, the majority of randomized controlled trials have failed to demonstrate benefit.[93] A recent meta-analysis of all randomized clinical trials of PPI versus placebo found a small benefit in favor of PPI; however, this was not statistically significant.[94] One potential reason for this may be the lack of a "gold standard" for the diagnosis of LPR. Inclusion criteria for these studies varied widely, as did the severity or symptoms, and not all studies relied on endoscopic laryngeal evaluation to assist in the diagnosis of LPR. It is therefore conceivable that some of these studies may have assigned diagnoses of LPR incorrectly. Thus, patients included in the treatment arms may not have truly suffered from LPR and diluted any actual treatment effect from PPIs.

Another confounding factor is confusion over proper PPI dosing for LPR treatment. Several investigators have demonstrated that once-daily PPI dosing (the standard for GERD therapy) has significant failure rates for LPR therapy.[95,96] One of the randomized clinical trials failing to show effect compared once daily pantoprazole to placebo in the treatment of LPR. This study demonstrated no difference in symptoms or endoscopic findings at 3 months between treatment and control groups.[97] This contrasts with the randomized controlled trial by El-Serag et al[92] which found significant improvement with BID lansoprazole therapy compared to placebo. More recently Park et al[88] demonstrated a response rate of 50% after 2 months of twice-daily PPI therapy compared to 28% on once-daily therapy. Additionally, 53% of nonresponders from the once-daily arm demonstrated improvement when switched to BID treatment.

Despite the contradictory findings from randomized controlled trials, the use of empiric PPI therapy remains the mainstay of first-line treatment for LPR. Many otolaryngologists favor twice-daily PPI therapy for moderate and severe LPR although the realities of insurance reimbursement for PPIs often stipulates a trial of once daily PPI.[15] This may underlie differences noted between academic and community ENT prescribing practices. Ahmed et al[55] reported that community otolaryngologists were more likely to initiate PPI therapy at once daily, compared to academic otolaryngologists who primarily initated therapy at twice daily. The importance of taking the PPI 20 to 30 minutes before meals must be stressed to the patient. Several authors have demonstrated that up to 54% of patients take PPIs improperly or suboptimally.[98–100] The pharmacokinetic properties of PPIs require activation of the target H^+-K^+ ATPase pump for efficient binding. Thus, taking a PPI 30 minutes before a meal allows absorption and circulation of the PPI to peak at the time of gastric H^+-K^+ ATPase stimulation. Additional recommendations include diet and behavioral modifications as discussed previously and summarized in Table 4–5. These interventions should be continued for a *minimum* of 3 months but in some individuals longer treatment periods are needed.[15] Less than 3-months empiric PPI therapy has been shown to produce no significant change in LPR symptoms compared to placebo,[87] while longer term therapy has been proven to be efficacious.[88] Further supporting the need for extended therapy, Belafksy et al[68] demonstrated that although a majority of LPR patients experience improvement of symptoms with 3 months PPI therapy, resolution of laryngeal injury as evidenced by erythema and edema can take 6 months to resolve.

In our practice, once a clinical diagnosis of LPR is made we initiate once daily PPI therapy and provide the patient with information regarding dietary and lifestyle changes. For those with significant anatomic findings such as airway stenosis, recurrent granulomas, or leukoplakia, as well as severe laryngospasm we begin with twice-daily treatment. Routine patients are seen at 2 month intervals and treatment response is followed by the RSI and RFS. Patients that experience partial or no response undergo further diagnostic evaluation, including esophageal manometry and 24-hour pH testing. We have found that empirically switching the brand of PPI has provided symptom relief in a portion of these patients. Changing medication within the PPI family has a strong theoretical foundation based on known heritable differences in cytochrome P450 (2C19) mediated metabolism of PPIs.[101–103] Prospective trials addressing the role of cytochrome P450 genotype testing in selecting PPI therapy are likely in the near future. Patients failing to respond to medication switching are escalated in PPI dosing to double-strength twice-daily therapy, and addition of a bedtime H2RA. Eventually we perform in-office TNE to evaluate for concurrent esophageal pathology as noted earlier.

It should be noted that some have raised the question of increased cancer risk among long-term PPI users, especially patients receiving high-dose therapy. In a large-scale cohort comparison, Yang et al[104] recently demonstrated no association with standard-dose PPI therapy and colorectal cancer. There was a nonsignificant trend towards increased risk among patients treated with high-dose PPI therapy ($p = 0.20$), however, that warrants judicious use of long-term high-dose PPI therapy. In our practice, once a patient experiences clinical *and endoscopic* improvement on PPI therapy (sometimes requiring 6 months or longer), the patient is gradually weaned from PPI therapy while maintaining lifestyle modifications. Bove et al[15] report a similar treatment paradigm, using an RSI <6 and

RFS <10 on two consecutive laryngoscopic examinations to determine appropriateness for PPI tapering. Patients are instructed to taper their PPI dosing to once daily, then once every other day, and then discontinue use. If their symptoms return they are escalated up on their PPI dosing. Similar to Bove et al[15] we have found a minority of LPR patients are able to tolerate complete discontinuation of PPI therapy.

Patients failing maximal medical therapy may require surgical evaluation and intervention in the form of laparoscopic Nissen-Rossetti fundoplication. This intervention holds particular appeal in light of the previously presented evidence for a nonacid component to at least some LPR.[14,20,105] Patients with an NAR contribution to their LPR would be expected to have persistent symptoms despite maximal acid-targeted medical therapy. There remain few medical options for the treatment of NAR. Some authors have advocated the use of baclofen, a γ-aminobutryic acid agonist, for the treatment of NAR.[106,107] In addition to this use being off-label, baclofen is associated with a number of undesirable side effects including nausea, drowsiness, and mental confusion.[108] Owing to these side effects, it is seldom employed for this use and surgical intervention remains the best option once antisecretory therapy has been maximized.

Some reports have indicated a relative lack of improvement for extraesophageal reflux treated with fundoplication.[109–111] Swoger et al[110] reported only 1 of 10 LPR patients recalcitrant to PPI therapy subsequently treated with fundoplication experienced symptom resolution. Similarly, So et al[111] reported that following fundoplication, patients were less likely to report relief of atypical symptoms (56%) compared to typical symptoms such as heartburn (93% of patients). However, when laryngeal symptoms alone were examined, 78% of patients reported improvement. Although no large-scale randomized clinical trials have (or likely ever will) address this question, the preponderance of evidence now appears to support a role for fundoplication in the management of recalcitrant LPR failing twice-daily PPI therapy.[112–117] Oelschlager et al[114] demonstrated a reduction in pharyngeal reflux from 7.9 to 1.6 episodes per 24 hours following laparoscopic fundoplication. These improvements are reflected in resolution of LPR symptoms as well. Rakita et al[116] recently reported up to 82% symptom improvement for patients with extraesophageal symptoms of GERD undergoing laparoscopic fundoplication. Similarly, Del Genio et al[113] report that of 1,000 patients undergoing laparoscopic fundoplication for GERD or LPR failing to respond to BID PPI therapy, 93% achieved symptom relief following surgical therapy. Most recently, Ogut et al[115] recently demonstrated an improvement in both RSI (from 25.5 to 16.5) and RFS (from 10.4 to 5.5) scores following fundoplication. Interestingly, preintervention testing using combined MII-pH may hold promise for predicting fundoplication success. Recently Mainie et al[118] found that 94% of patients with preoperative symptoms coincident with reflux were markedly improved or symptom-free at 14 months.

In summary, LPR is a complex disease of likely multifactorial etiology. The successful diagnosis and management of LPR patients requires careful collaboration across disciplinary lines. Future research is needed to elucidate the contributions of acidic and nonacidic reflux to LPR, and enhance our understanding of the pathophysiology of this disease process as well as the development of improved diagnostic modalities to select those patients most likely to respond to antireflux treatment.

REFERENCES

1. Koufman JA. Laryngopharyngeal reflux 2002: a new paradigm of airway disease. *Ear Nose Throat J.* 2002;81(9 suppl 2): 2-6.
2. Koufman JA, Amin MR, Panetti M. Prevalence of reflux in 113 consecutive patients with laryngeal and voice disorders. *Otolaryngol Head Neck Surg.* 2000;123(4):385-388.
3. Koufman JA. Laryngopharyngeal reflux is different from classic gastroesophageal reflux disease. *Ear Nose Throat J.* 2002;81(9 suppl 2):7-9.
4. Koufman JA. The otolaryngologic manifestations of gastroesophageal reflux disease (GERD): a clinical investigation of 225 patients using ambulatory 24-hour pH monitoring and an experimental investigation of the role of acid and pepsin in the development of laryngeal injury. *Laryngoscope.* 1991;101(4 pt 2, suppl 53):1-78.
5. Wiener GJ, Koufman JA, Wu WC, Cooper JB, Richter JE, Castell DO. Chronic hoarseness secondary to gastroesophageal reflux disease: documentation with 24-h ambulatory pH monitoring. *Am J Gastroenterol.* 1989; 84(12):1503-1508.
6. Postma GN, Tomek MS, Belafsky PC, Koufman JA. Esophageal motor function in laryngopharyngeal reflux is superior to that in classic gastroesophageal reflux disease. *Ann Otol Rhinol Laryngol.* 2001;110(12):1114-1116.
7. Koufman J, Sataloff RT, Toohill R. Laryngopharyngeal reflux: consensus conference report. *J Voice.* 1996;10(3): 215-216.
8. Lipan MJ, Reidenberg JS, Laitman JT. Anatomy of reflux: a growing health problem affecting structures of the head and neck. *Anat Rec B New Anat.* 2006;289(6):261-270.
9. Koufman JA, Aviv JE, Casiano RR, Shaw GY. Laryngopharyngeal reflux: position statement of the committee on speech, voice, and swallowing disorders of the American Academy of Otolaryngology-Head and Neck Surgery. *Otolaryngol Head Neck Surg.* 2002; 127(1):32-35.
10. Johnston N, Bulmer D, Gill GA, et al. Cell biology of laryngeal epithelial defenses in health and disease: further studies. *Ann Otol Rhinol Laryngol.* 2003;112(6):481-491.
11. Gill GA, Johnston N, Buda A, et al. Laryngeal epithelial defenses against laryngopharyngeal reflux: investigations of E-cadherin, carbonic anhydrase isoenzyme III, and pepsin. *Ann Otol Rhinol Laryngol.* 2005;114(12): 913-921.
12. Axford SE, Sharp N, Ross PE, et al. Cell biology of laryngeal epithelial defenses in health and disease: preliminary studies. *Ann Otol Rhinol Laryngol.* 2001; 110(12):1099-1108.
13. Charbel S, Khandwala F, Vaezi MF. The role of esophageal pH monitoring in symptomatic patients on PPI therapy. *Am J Gastroenterol.* 2005;100(2): 283-289.
14. Sasaki CT, Marotta J, Hundal J, Chow J, Eisen RN. Bile-induced laryngitis: is there a basis in evidence? *Ann Otol Rhinol Laryngol.* 2005;114(3):192-197.
15. Bove MJ, Rosen C. Diagnosis and management of laryngopharyngeal reflux disease. *Curr Opin Otolaryngol Head Neck Surg.* 2006;14(3):116-123.
16. Vela MF, Camacho-Lobato L, Srinivasan R, Tutuian R, Katz PO, Castell DO. Simultaneous intraesophageal impedance and pH measurement of acid and nonacid gastroesophageal reflux: effect

of omeprazole. *Gastroenterology.* 2001; 120(7):1599-1606.

17. Pellegrini CA, DeMeester TR, Wernly JA, Johnson LF, Skinner DB. Alkaline gastroesophageal reflux. *Am J Surg.* 1978;135(2):177-184.
18. Galli J, Calo L, Agostino S, et al. Bile reflux as possible risk factor in laryngopharyngeal inflammatory and neoplastic lesions. *Acta Otorhinolaryngol Ital.* 2003;23(5):377-382.
19. Shay S, Tutuian R, Sifrim D, et al. Twenty-four hour ambulatory simultaneous impedance and pH monitoring: a multicenter report of normal values from 60 healthy volunteers. *Am J Gastroenterol.* 2004;99(6):1037-1043.
20. Mainie I, Tutuian R, Shay S, et al. Acid and non-acid reflux in patients with persistent symptoms despite acid suppressive therapy: a multicentre study using combined ambulatory impedance-pH monitoring. *Gut.* 2006;55(10):1398-1402.
21. Reavis KM, Morris CD, Gopal DV, Hunter JG, Jobe BA. Laryngopharyngeal reflux symptoms better predict the presence of esophageal adenocarcinoma than typical gastroesophageal reflux symptoms. *Ann Surg.* 2004;239(6): 849-856; discussion 856-858.
22. Biacabe B, Gleich LL, Laccourreye O, Hartl DM, Bouchoucha M, Brasnu D. Silent gastroesophageal reflux disease in patients with pharyngolaryngeal cancer: further results. *Head Neck.* 1998;20(6):510-514.
23. Copper MP, Smit CF, Stanojcic LD, Devriese PP, Schouwenburg PF, Mathus-Vliegen LM. High incidence of laryngopharyngeal reflux in patients with head and neck cancer. *Laryngoscope.* 2000;110(6):1007-1011.
24. Cote DN, Miller RH. The association of gastroesophageal reflux and otolaryngologic disorders. *Compr Ther.* 1995; 21(2):80-84.
25. Qadeer MA, Colabianchi N, Strome M, Vaezi MF. Gastroesophageal reflux and laryngeal cancer: causation or association? A critical review. *Am J Otolaryngol.* 2006;27(2):119-128.
26. Vaezi MF, Qadeer MA, Lopez R, Colabianchi N. Laryngeal cancer and gastroesophageal reflux disease: a case-control study. *Am J Med.* 2006;119(9):768-776.
27. de Visser KE, Coussens LM. The inflammatory tumor microenvironment and its impact on cancer development. *Contrib Microbiol.* 2006;13:118-137.
28. Junankar SR, Eichten A, Kramer A, de Visser KE, Coussens LM. Analysis of immune cell infiltrates during squamous carcinoma development. *J Investig Dermatol Symp Proc.* 2006;11(1):36-43.
29. van Kempen LC, de Visser KE, Coussens LM. Inflammation, proteases and cancer. *Eur J Cancer.* 2006;42(6): 728-734.
30. Green BT, Broughton WA, O'Connor JB. Marked improvement in nocturnal gastroesophageal reflux in a large cohort of patients with obstructive sleep apnea treated with continuous positive airway pressure. *Arch Intern Med.* 2003;163(1):41-45.
31. Kasasbeh A, Kasasbeh E, Krishnaswamy G. Potential mechanisms connecting asthma, esophageal reflux, and obesity/sleep apnea complex—a hypothetical review. *Sleep Med Rev.* 2007; 11(1):47-58.
32. Shaheen NJ, Madanick RD, Alattar M, et al. Gastroesophageal reflux disease as an etiology of sleep disturbance in subjects with insomnia and minimal reflux symptoms: a pilot study of prevalence and response to therapy. *Dig Dis Sci.* 2008;53(6):1493-1499.
33. Valipour A, Makker HK, Hardy R, Emegbo S, Toma T, Spiro SG. Symptomatic gastroesophageal reflux in subjects with a breathing sleep disorder. *Chest.* 2002;121(6):1748-1753.
34. Wasilewska J, Kaczmarski M. Sleep-related breathing disorders in small children with nocturnal acid gastrooesophageal reflux. *Rocz Akad Med Bialymst.* 2004;49:98-102.

35. Wise SK, Wise JC, DelGaudio JM. Gastroesophageal reflux and laryngopharyngeal reflux in patients with sleep-disordered breathing. *Otolaryngol Head Neck Surg.* 2006;135(2):253–257.
36. Zanation AM, Senior BA. The relationship between extraesophageal reflux (EER) and obstructive sleep apnea (OSA). *Sleep Med Rev.* 2005;9(6):453–458.
37. DelGaudio JM. Direct nasopharyngeal reflux of gastric acid is a contributing factor in refractory chronic rhinosinusitis. *Laryngoscope.* 2005;115(6):946-957.
38. DiBaise JK, Huerter JV, Quigley EM. Sinusitis and gastroesophageal reflux disease. *Ann Intern Med.* 1998;129(12):1078.
39. Dibaise JK, Sharma VK. Does gastroesophageal reflux contribute to the development of chronic sinusitis? A review of the evidence. *Dis Esophagus.* 2006; 19(6):419-424.
40. Hamilos DL. Gastroesophageal reflux and sinusitis in asthma. *Clin Chest Med.* 1995;16(4):683-697.
41. Jecker P, Orloff LA, Wohlfeil M, Mann WJ. Gastroesophageal reflux disease (GERD), extraesophageal reflux (EER) and recurrent chronic rhinosinusitis. *Eur Arch Otorhinolaryngol.* 2006;263(7): 664-667.
42. Pincus RL, Kim HH, Silvers S, Gold S. A study of the link between gastric reflux and chronic sinusitis in adults. *Ear Nose Throat J.* 2006;85(3):174–178.
43. Ulualp SO, Toohill RJ, Hoffmann R, Shaker R. Possible relationship of gastroesophagopharyngeal acid reflux with pathogenesis of chronic sinusitis. *Am J Rhinol.* 1999;13(3):197–202.
44. Maronian NC, Azadeh H, Waugh P, Hillel A. Association of laryngopharyngeal reflux disease and subglottic stenosis. *Ann Otol Rhinol Laryngol.* 2001;110(7 pt 1):606–12.
45. Karkos PD, Leong SC, Apostolidou MT, Apostolidis T. Laryngeal manifestations and pediatric laryngopharyngeal reflux. *Am J Otolaryngol.* 2006;27(3):200–203.
46. Lorenz RR. Adult laryngotracheal stenosis: etiology and surgical management. *Curr Opin Otolaryngol Head Neck Surg.* 2003;11(6):467–472.
47. Olson NR. Laryngopharyngeal manifestations of gastroesophageal reflux disease. *Otolaryngol Clin North Am.* 1991;24(5):1201–1213.
48. Roh JL, Lee YW, Park HT. Effect of acid, pepsin, and bile acid on the stenotic progression of traumatized subglottis. *Am J Gastroenterol.* 2006;101(6): 1186–1192.
49. Toohill RJ, Ulualp SO, Shaker R. Evaluation of gastroesophageal reflux in patients with laryngotracheal stenosis. *Ann Otol Rhinol Laryngol.* 1998; 107(12):1010–1014.
50. Morse CA, Quan SF, Mays MZ, Green C, Stephen G, Fass R. Is there a relationship between obstructive sleep apnea and gastroesophageal reflux disease? *Clin Gastroenterol Hepatol.* 2004;2(9): 761–768.
51. Friedman M, Gurpinar B, Lin HC, Schalch P, Joseph NJ. Impact of treatment of gastroesophageal reflux on obstructive sleep apnea-hypopnea syndrome. *Ann Otol Rhinol Laryngol.* 2007;116(11): 805–811.
52. Book DT, Rhee JS, Toohill RJ, Smith TL. Perspectives in laryngopharyngeal reflux: an international survey. *Laryngoscope.* 2002;112(8 pt 1):1399–1406.
53. Vaezi MF, Hicks DM, Abelson TI, Richter JE. Laryngeal signs and symptoms and gastroesophageal reflux disease (GERD): a critical assessment of cause and effect association. *Clin Gastroenterol Hepatol.* 2003;1(5):333–344.
54. Ford CN. Evaluation and management of laryngopharyngeal reflux. *JAMA.* 2005;294(12):1534–1540.
55. Ahmed TF, Khandwala F, Abelson TI, et al. Chronic laryngitis associated with gastroesophageal reflux: prospective assessment of differences in practice patterns between gastroenterologists

and ENT physicians. *Am J Gastroenterol.* 2006;101(3):470-478.

56. Belafsky PC, Postma GN, Koufman JA. Validity and reliability of the reflux symptom index (RSI). *J Voice.* 2002; 16(2):274-277.
57. Mesallam TA, Stemple JC, Sobeih TM, Elluru RG. Reflux symptom index versus reflux finding score. *Ann Otol Rhinol Laryngol.* 2007;116(6):436-440.
58. Belafsky PC, Postma GN, Koufman JA. The validity and reliability of the reflux finding score (RFS). *Laryngoscope.* 2001;111(8):1313-1317.
59. Gaynor EB. Laryngeal complications of GERD. *J Clin Gastroenterol.* 2000;30 (3 suppl):S31-S34.
60. Qadeer MA, Swoger J, Milstein C, et al. Correlation between symptoms and laryngeal signs in laryngopharyngeal reflux. *Laryngoscope.* 2005;115(11): 1947-1952.
61. Ylitalo R, Lindestad PA, Ramel S. Symptoms, laryngeal findings, and 24-hour pH monitoring in patients with suspected gastroesophago-pharyngeal reflux. *Laryngoscope.* 2001;111(10):1735-1741.
62. Hickson C, Simpson CB, Falcon R. Laryngeal pseudosulcus as a predictor of laryngopharyngeal reflux. *Laryngoscope.* 2001;111(10):1742-1745.
63. Belafsky PC, Postma GN, Koufman JA. The association between laryngeal pseudosulcus and laryngopharyngeal reflux. *Otolaryngol Head Neck Surg.* 2002;126(6):649-652.
64. Ylitalo R, Ramel S. Extraesophageal reflux in patients with contact granuloma: a prospective controlled study. *Ann Otol Rhinol Laryngol.* 2002;111(5 pt 1):441-446.
65. Hill RK, Simpson CB, Velazquez R, Larson N. Pachydermia is not diagnostic of active laryngopharyngeal reflux disease. *Laryngoscope.* 2004;114(9):1557-1561.
66. Hicks DM, Ours TM, Abelson TI, Vaezi MF, Richter JE. The prevalence of hypopharynx findings associated with gastroesophageal reflux in normal volunteers. *J Voice.* 2002;16(4):564-579.
67. Milstein CF, Charbel S, Hicks DM, Abelson TI, Richter JE, Vaezi MF. Prevalence of laryngeal irritation signs associated with reflux in asymptomatic volunteers: impact of endoscopic technique (rigid vs. flexible laryngoscope). *Laryngoscope.* 2005;115(12):2256-2261.
68. Belafsky PC, Postma GN, Koufman JA. Laryngopharyngeal reflux symptoms improve before changes in physical findings. *Laryngoscope.* 2001;111(6): 979-981.
69. Vaezi MF. Laryngitis and gastroesophageal reflux disease: increasing prevalence or poor diagnostic tests? *Am J Gastroenterol.* 2004;99(5):786-788.
70. Shaker R, Bardan E, Gu C, Kern M, Torrico L, Toohill R. Intrapharyngeal distribution of gastric acid refluxate. *Laryngoscope.* 2003;113(7):1182-1191.
71. Ulualp SO, Toohill RJ, Hoffmann R, Shaker R. Pharyngeal pH monitoring in patients with posterior laryngitis. *Otolaryngol Head Neck Surg.* 1999;120(5): 672-677.
72. Ulualp SO, Toohill RJ, Shaker R. Pharyngeal acid reflux in patients with single and multiple otolaryngologic disorders. *Otolaryngol Head Neck Surg.* 1999; 121(6):725-730.
73. Oelschlager BK, Eubanks TR, Maronian N, et al. Laryngoscopy and pharyngeal pH are complementary in the diagnosis of gastroesophageal-laryngeal reflux. *J Gastrointest Surg.* 2002;6(2):189-194.
74. Shaker R, Milbrath M, Ren J, et al. Esophagopharyngeal distribution of refluxed gastric acid in patients with reflux laryngitis. *Gastroenterology.* 1995;109(5):1575-1582.
75. Sermon F, Vanden Brande S, Roosens B, Mana F, Deron P, Urbain D. Is ambulatory 24-h dual-probe pH monitoring useful in suspected ENT manifestations of GERD? *Dig Liver Dis.* 2004;36(2): 105-110.

76. Postma GN, Belafsky PC, Aviv JE, Koufman JA. Laryngopharyngeal reflux testing. *Ear Nose Throat J.* 2002;81(9 suppl 2):14–18.
77. Merati AL, Lim HJ, Ulualp SO, Toohill RJ. Meta-analysis of upper probe measurements in normal subjects and patients with laryngopharyngeal reflux. *Ann Otol Rhinol Laryngol.* 2005;114(3): 177–182.
78. Dobhan R, Castell DO. Normal and abnormal proximal esophageal acid exposure: results of ambulatory dual-probe pH monitoring. *Am J Gastroenterol.* 1993;88(1):25–29.
79. Tutuian R, Vela MF, Shay SS, Castell DO. Multichannel intraluminal impedance in esophageal function testing and gastroesophageal reflux monitoring. *J Clin Gastroenterol.* 2003;37(3):206–215.
80. Eckley CA, Michelsohn N, Rizzo LV, Tadokoro CE, Costa HO. Salivary epidermal growth factor concentration in adults with reflux laryngitis. *Otolaryngol Head Neck Surg.* 2004;131(4):401–406.
81. Johnston N, Dettmar PW, Lively MO, et al. Effect of pepsin on laryngeal stress protein (Sep70, Sep53, and Hsp70) response: role in laryngopharyngeal reflux disease. *Ann Otol Rhinol Laryngol.* 2006;115(1):47–58.
82. Johnston N, Knight J, Dettmar PW, Lively MO, Koufman J. Pepsin and carbonic anhydrase isoenzyme III as diagnostic markers for laryngopharyngeal reflux disease. *Laryngoscope.* 2004; 114(12):2129–2134.
83. Knight J, Lively MO, Johnston N, Dettmar PW, Koufman JA. Sensitive pepsin immunoassay for detection of laryngopharyngeal reflux. *Laryngoscope.* 2005;115(8):1473–1478.
84. Katz PO. State of the art: extraesophageal manifestations of gastroesophageal reflux disease. *Rev Gastroenterol Disord.* 2005;5(3):126–134.
85. Fackler WK, Ours TM, Vaezi MF, Richter JE. Long-term effect of H2RA therapy on nocturnal gastric acid breakthrough. *Gastroenterology.* 2002;122(3):625–632.
86. Katz PO. Medical therapy for gastroesophageal reflux disease in 2007. *Rev Gastroenterol Disord.* 2007;7(4): 193–203.
87. Steward DL, Wilson KM, Kelly DH, et al. Proton pump inhibitor therapy for chronic laryngo-pharyngitis: a randomized placebo-control trial. *Otolaryngol Head Neck Surg.* 2004;131(4):342–350.
88. Park W, Hicks DM, Khandwala F, et al. Laryngopharyngeal reflux: prospective cohort study evaluating optimal dose of proton-pump inhibitor therapy and pretherapy predictors of response. *Laryngoscope.* 2005;115(7):1230–1238.
89. Klopocka M, Sinkiewicz A, Budzynski J, Pulkowski G, Swiatkowski M. Improvement in clinical course and laryngeal appearance in selected patients with chronic laryngitis after eight weeks of therapy with rabeprazole. *Med Sci Monit.* 2004;10(10):PI115–P118.
90. Vaezi MF. Extraesophageal manifestations of gastroesophageal reflux disease. *Clin Cornerstone.* 2003;5(4):32–38; discussion 39–40.
91. Shaw GY, Searl JP. Laryngeal manifestations of gastroesophageal reflux before and after treatment with omeprazole. *South Med J.* 1997;90(11):1115–1122.
92. El-Serag HB, Lee P, Buchner A, Inadomi JM, Gavin M, McCarthy DM. Lansoprazole treatment of patients with chronic idiopathic laryngitis: a placebo-controlled trial. *Am J Gastroenterol.* 2001;96(4): 979–983.
93. Vaezi MF, Richter JE, Stasney CR, et al. Treatment of chronic posterior laryngitis with esomeprazole. *Laryngoscope.* 2006;116(2):254–260.
94. Qadeer MA, Phillips CO, Rocio Lopez A, et al. Proton pump inhibitor therapy for suspected GERD-related chronic laryngitis: a meta-analysis of randomized controlled trials. *Clin Otolaryngol.* 2008;33(2):113.

95. Leite LP, Johnston BT, Just RJ, Castell DO. Persistent acid secretion during omeprazole therapy: a study of gastric acid profiles in patients demonstrating failure of omeprazole therapy. *Am J Gastroenterol.* 1996;91(8):1527-1531.
96. Amin MR, Postma GN, Johnson P, Digges N, Koufman JA. Proton pump inhibitor resistance in the treatment of laryngopharyngeal reflux. *Otolaryngol Head Neck Surg.* 2001;125(4):374-378.
97. Wo JM, Koopman J, Harrell SP, Parker K, Winstead W, Lentsch E. Double-blind, placebo-controlled trial with single-dose pantoprazole for laryngopharyngeal reflux. *Am J Gastroenterol.* 2006; 101(9):1972-1978; quiz 2169.
98. Chheda NN, Postma GN. Patient compliance with proton pump inhibitor therapy in an otolaryngology practice. *Ann Otol Rhinol Laryngol.* 2008;117(9): 670-672.
99. Hungin AP, Rubin G, O'Flanagan H. Factors influencing compliance in long-term proton pump inhibitor therapy in general practice. *Br J Gen Pract.* 1999; 49(443):463-464.
100. Gunaratnam NT, Jessup TP, Inadomi J, Lascewski DP. Sub-optimal proton pump inhibitor dosing is prevalent in patients with poorly controlled gastro-oesophageal reflux disease. *Aliment Pharmacol Ther.* 2006;23(10):1473-1477.
101. Furuta T, Shirai N, Sugimoto M, Ohashi K, Ishizaki T. Pharmacogenomics of proton pump inhibitors. *Pharmacogenomics.* 2004;5(2):181-202.
102. Fock KM, Ang TL, Bee LC, Lee EJ. Proton pump inhibitors: do differences in pharmacokinetics translate into differences in clinical outcomes? *Clin Pharmacokinet.* 2008;47(1):1-6.
103. Sugimoto M, Furuta T, Shirai N, Ikuma M, Hishida A, Ishizaki T. Initial 48-hour acid inhibition by intravenous infusion of omeprazole, famotidine, or both in relation to cytochrome P450 2C19 genotype status. *Clin Pharmacol Ther.* 2006;80(5):539-548.
104. Yang YX, Hennessy S, Propert K, Hwang WT, Sedarat A, Lewis JD. Chronic proton pump inhibitor therapy and the risk of colorectal cancer. *Gastroenterology.* 2007;133(3):748-754.
105. Tutuian R, Mainie I, Agrawal A, Adams D, Castell DO. Nonacid reflux in patients with chronic cough on acid-suppressive therapy. *Chest.* 2006;130(2):386-391.
106. Koek GH, Sifrim D, Lerut T, Janssens J, Tack J. Effect of the GABA(B) agonist baclofen in patients with symptoms and duodeno-gastro-oesophageal reflux refractory to proton pump inhibitors. *Gut.* 2003;52(10):1397-1402.
107. Vela MF, Tutuian R, Katz PO, Castell DO. Baclofen decreases acid and non-acid post-prandial gastro-oesophageal reflux measured by combined multichannel intraluminal impedance and pH. *Aliment Pharmacol Ther.* 2003; 17(2):243-251.
108. Leung NY, Whyte IM, Isbister GK. Baclofen overdose: defining the spectrum of toxicity. *Emerg Med Australas.* 2006;18(1):77-82.
109. Bresadola V, Dado G, Favero A, Terrosu G, Barriga Sainz M, Bresadola F. Surgical therapy for patients with extraesophageal symptoms of gastroesophageal reflux disease. *Minerva Chir.* 2006; 61(1):9-15.
110. Swoger J, Ponsky J, Hicks DM, et al. Surgical fundoplication in laryngopharyngeal reflux unresponsive to aggressive acid suppression: a controlled study. *Clin Gastroenterol Hepatol.* 2006;4(4): 433-441.
111. So JB, Zeitels SM, Rattner DW. Outcomes of atypical symptoms attributed to gastroesophageal reflux treated by laparoscopic fundoplication. *Surgery.* 1998;124(1):28-32.
112. Westcott CJ, Hopkins MB, Bach K, Postma GN, Belafsky PC, Koufman JA. Fundoplication for laryngopharyngeal

reflux disease. *J Am Coll Surg.* 2004; 199(1):23-30.

113. Del Genio G, Rossetti G, Brusciano L, et al. Laparoscopic Nissen-Rossetti fundoplication is effective to control gastro-oesophageal and pharyngeal reflux detected using 24-hour oesophageal impedance and pH monitoring (MII-pH). *Acta Otorhinolaryngol Ital.* 2006; 26(5):287-292.
114. Oelschlager BK, Eubanks TR, Oleynikov D, Pope C, Pellegrini CA. Symptomatic and physiologic outcomes after operative treatment for extraesophageal reflux. *Surg Endosc.* 2002;16(7):1032-1036.
115. Ogut F, Ersin S, Engin EZ, et al. The effect of laparoscopic Nissen fundoplication on laryngeal findings and voice quality. *Surg Endosc.* 2007;21(4):549-554.
116. Rakita S, Villadolid D, Thomas A, et al. Laparoscopic Nissen fundoplication offers high patient satisfaction with relief of extraesophageal symptoms of gastroesophageal reflux disease. *Am Surg.* 2006;72(3):207-212.
117. Lindstrom DR, Wallace J, Loehrl TA, Merati AL, Toohill RJ. Nissen fundoplication surgery for extraesophageal manifestations of gastroesophageal reflux (EER). *Laryngoscope.* 2002;112(10): 1762-1765.
118. Mainie I, Tutuian R, Agrawal A, Adams D, Castell DO. Combined multichannel intraluminal impedance-pH monitoring to select patients with persistent gastro-oesophageal reflux for laparoscopic Nissen fundoplication. *Br J Surg.* 2006; 93(12):1483-1487.

5

Laryngopharyngeal Reflux and Laryngeal Disorders: The Role of the Speech-Language Pathologist

Thomas Murry, Sabrina Cukier-Blaj, and Douglas M. Hicks

LARYNGOPHARYNGEAL REFLUX

Introduction

The presence of acid in the lower esophagus resulting in symptoms such as heartburn, regurgitation, or burping is a common occurrence after a meal and it occurs in most people occasionally. Laryngopharyngeal reflux (LPR) refers to the backflow of stomach contents passing through the upper esophageal area into the hypopharynx and causing laryngeal edema and hoarseness. Not all symptoms of gastroesophageal reflux (GER) are associated with LPR; in fact, the symptoms, types of patients and treatments for these two conditions are quite different. Patients with LPR complain of predominant head and neck issues rather than traditional gastric issues. They usually do not have prolonged periods of acid exposure and they do not have esophageal dysmotility and prolonged esophageal acid clearance times. GER patients have a much higher incidence of prolonged acid clearance times than LPR patients and may be more likely to have esophageal dysmotility.[1]

The primary defect in GER is lower esophageal dysfunction. In LPR, there is a concomitant upper esophageal sphincter dysfunction. The laryngeal symptoms seen in LPR require specialized testing and treatment. LPR has been reported to be associated with subglottic stenosis, laryngeal carcinoma, polypoid degeneration, laryngospasm, paradoxic vocal fold movement, and vocal fold nodules.[1] Testing is frequently done by otolaryngologists (as reported in Chapter 4), and a speech-language pathologist will eventually see patients for both specialized endoscopy and treatment for dysphonia. Once the medical diagnosis and pharmacological prescriptions are offered by the otolaryngologist, the high incidence of hoarseness, voice strain, and other laryngeal findings in patients with LPR require rehabilitation of the vocal mechanism by a speech-language professional who specializes in voice disorders. The otolaryngologist and speech-language pathologist make up the management team to restore the voice and swallowing of the patient with LPR so that he or she may return to normal function.

This is usually done in conjunction with the gastroenterologist who may also be involved in medical management if lower esophageal symptoms are present.

Symptoms

Patients with LPR have as major complaints hoarseness and/or voice loss, sensation of something in the throat (globus), difficulty swallowing (dysphagia), cough, chronic throat clearing, and sore throat.[1-5] Table 5-1 presents the common symptoms and their prevalence in a group of patients seen at Columbia University Medical Center. The findings are similar to those reported by others.[1,2] The worst complaints were throat clearing, throat mucus, hoarseness, and cough.

Table 5–1. Common Symptoms in a Cohort of 70 Consecutive Patients with Laryngeal Findings of LPR and PVFM

Symptoms	%
Throat clearing	80
Throat mucus	74,3
Hoarseness	68,6
Annoying cough	62,9
Something sticking in the throat	54,3
Breathing difficulties	48,6
Coughing after lying down	42,9
Heartburn/chest pain	42,9
Difficulty swallowing	28,6

Voice and Laryngeal Conditions Associated with LPR

Functional Dysphonia

Functional dysphonia is the impairment of voice production in the absence of structural change or neurogenic disease of the larynx. Delineation of functional dysphonia is based on medical history, laryngoscopic, perceptual-acoustic, musculoskeletal, and psychological features. Patients with muscular tension dysphonia (MTD), a kind of functional dysphonia, often have an associated history of gastroesophageal reflux and tobacco use.[3] The clinical findings by the speech pathologists are hoarse voice quality, poor breath support, inappropriate pitch and visible cervical tension.[6]

Edema and Other Benign Lesions

The high incidence of hoarseness and vocal fatigue in patients with diagnosed LPR is related to the presence of abnormal findings in the visual examination of the larynx with endoscopic evaluation. Endoscopy of the larynx and vocal folds may be done in real time with standard flexible endoscopy or with videostrobolaryngoscopy, a technique that allows slow motion observation of the rapid vibratory movements of the vocal folds. The abnormal videostroboscopic findings in patients with LPR are: vocal fold edema, asymmetry of the mucous layer, vessel dilation, and lack of complete vocal fold closure (Color Plate 5). Regarding the pathognomic laryngeal findings related to LPR, Ylitalo[7] found that posterior laryngitis occurs in up to 70% of LPR patients. It is characterized by edema, hypertrophy, and sometimes erythema and hyperemia on the posterior wall of the glottis. Furthermore, diffuse vocal fold edema, infraglottic edema reaching from the anterior commissure to the posterior wall, also referred to as *pseudosulcus*, and vocal fold granuloma are strongly associated with LPR.[2,8,9]

However, it is important to note that in a cohort of 105 normal subjects, nearly 80% were found to have an interarytenoid bar or posterior commissure hypertrophy.[7] Thus, LPR may be found with a multitude of signs and symptoms. Voice use as well as acid injury must be considered when examining the vocal folds.

Polypoid degeneration is a less common finding that represents a chronic process of laryngeal inflammation associated with acid injury to the vocal folds. It presents usually in both vocal folds and occurs most often in women who smoke.

Vocal Process Granuloma

Vocal process granuloma is a noncancerous growth that appears on one or both vocal processes of the arytenoid cartilage. It is comprised of cells and substances often found in sites of inflammation and reflects a response to irritation or injury. Granulomas may be quite small and cause the patient to cough or clear his throat occasionally. They may also be large and in multiples that cause breathing difficulties, severe voice changes, and difficulty or pain when swallowing. Granulomas on the vocal process are often seen in patients with LPR and may also be found in patients following traumatic intubation and in patients who continuously use a tight strained voice (Color Plate 6).

Historically, granulomas were treated with laryngeal surgery; however, there was a high incidence of recurrence. Proper treatment requires the combination of behavioral and pharmacologic assessments.

Carcinoma of the Larynx

The most important risk factors for the development of laryngeal carcinoma are tobacco and alcohol use, but LPR also appears to be an important corisk factor, especially in nonsmokers. Koufman[9] reported 31 consecutive cases of laryngeal carcinoma. LPR was documented in 84% of the cases, but only 58% overall were active smokers. The exact relationship between LPR and malignant degeneration remains unknown, but the available pH-metry data suggest that most patients who develop laryngeal malignancy both smoke and have LPR. In addition, leukoplakia and other premalignant appearing lesions may be related to the presence of LPR and result in dysphonia.[10,11]

Paradoxic Vocal Fold Motion

Paradoxic vocal fold motion (PVFM), also known as vocal cord dysfunction (VCD) is a condition characterized by the intermittent adduction of the vocal folds during quiet breathing and/or following speaking. The most common symptoms are dyspnea, cough, and dysphonia. The etiology is related to laryngopharyngeal reflux and loss of laryngeal sensation.[12,13] It can be also related to allergies, inhaled asthma, and their medications. It is hypothesized that paradoxic vocal fold adduction may be accentuated due to the mechanical stimulation or chemical irritation of the laryngeal mucosa (due to LPR), such that various extrinsic stimuli trigger reflexive closure of the vocal folds at pathologically low thresholds. Recent reports of patients diagnosed with PVFM indicate the presence of LPR ranging from 35% to as high as 90%.[12,14]

Laryngospasm

Laryngospasm is a serious condition defined as a sudden-onset, rapid, and forceful contraction of the laryngeal sphincter resulting in airway obstruction or complete glottic closure, and *apnea* (temporary suspension of breathing) with duration up to 20 seconds. Laryngospasms occur in response to a noxious stimulus and may represent an abnormal excitation and/or loss of inhibition of the laryngeal closure reflex. The pathophysiology of laryngospasm may be related to LPR, upper respiratory infection, and cough. Similar to PVFM, it is hypothesized that cough increases the refluxate that contacts the posterior cricoid area and spills into the larynx. This noxious stimulus triggers the vagal reflex that often results in laryngospasm.[15] Episodic laryngospasm subsides following antireflux therapy and may be the only treatment necessary for this problem.[16] Excessive episodic laryngospasm coupled with cough and choking may lead to dysphonia requiring management by a laryngologist and speech-language pathologist.

Dysphagia

Dysphagia is an abnormality of swallowing. Patients with LPR usually have swallowing symptoms such as food sticking, difficulty with swallowing pills, and excessive swallowing of saliva. Moreover, Aviv et al[17] reported that patients with LPR often have a moderate to severe sensory reduction of the laryngeal adductor reflex (LAR)[17,18] implying that there is a high possibility of silent aspiration. Pharmacological treatment with proton-pump inhibitor (PPI) was shown to improve the response of sensation in patients with LPR.[17,19]

ROLE OF THE SLP

Introduction

The high incidence of voice disorders in patients with LPR is the basis for the voice specialist to be part of the management team. Figure 5-1 shows the management of a patient with LPR and voice disorder. Table 5-2 summarizes the common treatments for LPR, many involving direct voice therapy.

The speech-language pathologist (SLP) diagnostic procedures consist of a comprehensive voice use profile, health history, functional voice assessment, laryngeal visualization, and eventual treatments recommendations. Important questions related to the voice usage are: the patient's profession (if he is a professional voice user), special complaints such as voice fatigue, loss of voice after some period of talking, and vocal instability during the day. The history of the voice problem should also be investigated, as it relates to the duration of the problem, circumstances surrounding the onset of the problem, previous voice problems and treatments, current versus onset profile, and how the voice problem affects the

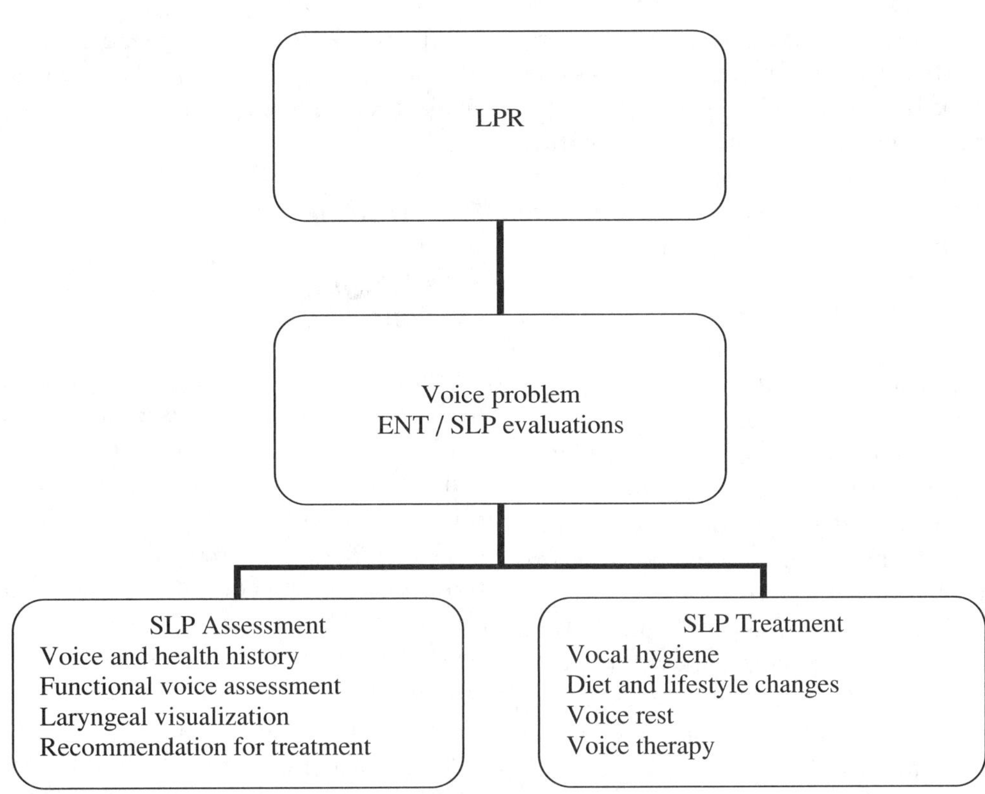

Fig 5–1. Speech-language pathologist management of patients with laryngopharyngeal reflux (LPR) and voice disorders.

Table 5–2. Most Common Treatments of Voice Disorders Associated with Laryngopharyngeal Reflux (LPR)

Common Disorders	Treatments	
	SLP	**Laryngeal Surgery**
Functional dysphonia	VH + VT	No
Edema and other benign lesions	VH + VT*	Depends on the lesion
Polypoid degeneration	VH + VT*	Often
Vocal process granuloma	VH + VT	Rare
Carcinoma of the larynx	VH + VT	Surgery, chemotherapy, and radiotherapy
Paradoxic vocal fold motion	VH + VT	No
Laryngospasm	VH	No
Dysphagia associated to reflux	VH	Depending on findings

Vocal hygiene and changes in diet and lifestyle (VH).
Voice therapy (VT).
*Pre and postsurgery.

patient's work and social status. Here, standardized assessment tools such as the Voice Handicap Index (VHI),[20] VHI-10,[21] and Voice Activity and Participation Profile (VAPP)[23] may be helpful in completing the voice assessment related to quality of life and the patient's perceived voice severity.

The health history involves survey for smoking, alcohol use, and consumption of specific foods such as those containing caffeine or mint. The presence of concomitant diseases, exposure to other irritant airways (allergies, asthma medications, chemical perfumes and air pollution), and the use of medications are also important.

The presence of acoustic, physiologic and perceptual abnormalities of the voice and impairment of the patient's quality of life suggest SLP treatment, concomitant to the pharmacologic care.

Diagnosis

The diagnosis of LPR can be strongly suggested by reflux symptoms, such as hoarseness, cough and throat clearing, and physical laryngeal examination findings. There are pathognomic findings of LPR, seen on transnasal flexible laryngoscopy examination and videostroboscopy that were described above. Further testing known as sensory test is also helpful in diagnosis. It is a calibrated air pulse delivered to the aryepiglottic fold region of the larynx that identifies the laryngeal adductor reflex (LAR). The LAR pressure threshold has previously been categorized according to normal, moderate, and severely reduced sensation.

The combination of patient history, physical examination, and laryngeal sensory testing has been demonstrated to be as effective as the double-probe 24-hour pH monitoring to diagnose laryngopharyngeal reflux disease.[23,24]

SLP Treatments

Vocal Hygiene and Changes in Diet and Lifestyle

Vocal hygiene programs are addressed to prevent vocal abuse. It is important to explain to the patient how the voice is produced and what is traumatic or stressful to the vocal folds.

The orientation to reduce or eliminate throat clearing and cough is common and necessary for the success of the treatment. Vocal performers need specific counseling to address their extraordinary voice demands. Hydration is a key aspect of any vocal hygiene program. It includes an increase of water consumption, steam inhalation, attention to humidity of the ambient air, and administration of mucolitics to thin the phlegm. Simply by increasing the act of swallowing, the patient may reduce the sensation of excess phlegm and throat clearing.

Changes in diet and lifestyle are also addressed and monitored. Patients with LPR should reduce or avoid dry ambient air, tobacco, alcohol, caffeinated beverages, as well as mint, and antihistaminic agents.

Voice Rest and Conservation

Counseling regarding voice rest and conservation is appropriate when there is a high degree of laryngeal inflammation. Voice rest refers to the complete cessation of voicing and is addressed only in extreme situations, such as acute laryngitis or laryngeal trauma. Voice conservation refers to modified voice use such as reduced loud talking, singing, and extensive conversations. The outcome of voice conservation usually results in enough positive change to promote tissue recovery that will lead to voice improvement. Long-term establishment and maintenance of new, vocally healthy habits are best formed in the very activities or settings that previously fostered abuse.[25]

Voice Therapy

The growing body of research in vocal fold physiology and voice disorders has increased the understanding of techniques and methods for behavioral management of voice disorders as well as their efficacious use.

The SLP uses behavioral management techniques to reduce traumatic voice use, increase vocal efficiency, and produce a clearer tone. Cognitive strategies and perceptual cues are also used for acquisition of motor skills and monitoring voice quality.[26]

The various voice disorders related to LPR include functional dysphonia, muscle tension dysphonia (MTD), granuloma, benign and malignant lesions, and PVFM (see Table 5-2). Many of these respond well to voice therapy provided by the speech-language pathologist. The specifics of vocal therapy will be guided according to the pathophysiology, function, and perceptual and acoustics parameters of the voice disorder.

Treatment of Vocal Hyperfunction

Vocal hyperfunction is common in patients with MTD, granuloma, and benign lesions. Clinical findings are hoarse voice quality, poor breath support, inappropriate pitch, and visible cervical tension.[27]

Voice therapy to reduce vocal hyperfunction can be addressed by vocal function exercises, resonant voice therapy, confidential voice therapy, and a variety of muscle tension unloading techniques. The goal of the techniques is to retrain muscle patterns to produce the clearest and most prominent voice with less effort and most efficiency of voice use.

Different techniques are addressed according to the voice quality assessment and physiology description. The usual eligible techniques are training airflow during phonation, facilitators for oral resonance, and using variations in intensity and frequency.

Treatment for Breathing and Cough

The presence of cough, PVFM, and laryngospasm has been behaviorally treated with a respiratory retraining program. It consists of a series of breathing exercises that focus on breathing with minimal expiratory force and with a regular rhythm. Originally reported by Christopher et al,[28] the exercises begin with the patient standing comfortably or walking slowly and exhaling without forceful inhaling. As the patient develops a steady rhythm, resistance to breathing out is increased by having the patient produce sounds such as "sh" or "s." Eventually, the patient develops an effortless, rhythmic breathing pattern and learns to avoid sudden inspiratory bursts that interrupt the normal breathing pattern.[12,14,28,29]

An education component is also part of the treatment and emphasizes the futility and negative side effects of repeated coughing; the benefits of cough suppression, and the capacity of individuals to develop voluntary control over cough. The cough suppression component required participants to anticipate when a cough was about to occur and then implement a strategy to suppress or replace it.

SUMMARY

Laryngopharyngeal reflux is commonly associated with laryngeal and voice disorders. The patient's main complaints are hoarseness, throat clearing, excess throat mucus, choking, and cough. The diagnosis is based on history and specialized laryngoscopic assessments. A series of concomitant lesions and disorders are described, such as functional dysphonia, benign vocal fold lesions, and paradoxic vocal fold motion. The role of the speech-language pathologist is to manage the assessment and treatment of the patient with LPR and voice disorders. Vocal hygiene programs, voice conservation counseling and proper voice therapy are addressed according to physiologic, perceptual, and acoustics vocal assessments. However, the key for the success of the patient care is a multidisciplinary approach involving the gastroenterologist, otolaryngologist, and a speech-language pathologist who specializes in voice disorders.

REFERENCES

1. Belafsky PC, Postma GN, Amin MR, Koufman JA. Symptoms and findings of laryngopharyngeal reflux. *Ear Nose Throat J.* 2002;81(9 suppl 2):10–13.
2. Belafsky PC, Postma GN, Koufman JA. The validity and reliability of the reflux finding score (RFS). *Laryngoscope.* 2001; 111(8):1313–1317.
3. Tauber S, Gross M, Issing WJ. Association of laryngopharyngeal symptoms with gastroesophageal reflux disease. *Laryngoscope.* 2002;112:879–886.
4. Vaezi MF, Hicks DM, Abelson TI, Richter JE. Laryngeal signs and symptoms and gastroesophageal reflux disease (GERD): a critical assessment of cause and effect association. *Clin Gastroenterol Hepatol.* 2003;1:333–344.
5. Qadeer MA, Swoger J, Milstein C, et al. Correlation between symptoms and laryngeal signs in laryngopharyngeal reflux. *Laryngoscope.* 2005;115:1947–1952.
6. Karkos PD, Yates PD, Carding PN, Wilson JA. Is laryngopharyngeal reflux related to functional dysphonia? *Ann Otol Rhinol Laryngol.* 2007;116(1):24–29.
7. Ylitalo R. Reflux and the larynx. Merati AL, Bielamowicz SA, eds. In: *Textbook of Voice Disorders.* San Diego, Calif: Plural Publishing, 2007.
8. Koufman JA. The otolaryngologic manifestations of gastroesophageal reflux disease (GERD): a clinical investigation of 225 patients using ambulatory 24-hour pH monitoring and an experimental investigation of the role of acid and pepsin in the development of laryngeal injury. *Laryngoscope.* 1991;101(53),1–78.
9. Koufman JA, Aviv JE, Casiano RR, Shaw GY. Laryngopharyngeal reflux: position statement of the committee on speech, voice, and swallowing disorders of the American Academy of Otolaryngology-Head and Neck Surgery. *Otolaryngol Head Neck Surg.* 2002;127(1), 32–35.
10. Hicks DM, Ours TM, Abelson TI, Vaezi MF, Richter JE. The prevalence of hypopharynx findings associated with gastroesophageal reflux in normal volunteers. *J Voice.* 2002;16(4):564–579.
11. Koufman JA, Burke AJ. The etiology and pathogenesis of laryngeal carcinoma. *Otolaryngol Clin North Am.* 1997;30(1): 1–19.
12. Murry T, Tabaee A, Oxczarzak V, Aviv JE. Respiratory retraining therapy and man-

agement of laryngopharyngeal reflux in the treatment of patients with cough and paradoxical vocal fold movement disorder. *Ann Otol Rhinol Laryngol.* 2006;115(10):754-758.

13. Andrianopoulos MV, Gallivan GJ, Gallivan KH. PVCM, PVCD, EPL and irritable larynx syndrome: what are we talking about and how do we treat it? *J Voice.* 2000;14(4): 607-618.
14. Vertigan AE, Theodoros DG, Gibson PG, Winkworth AL. Efficacy of speech pathology management for chronic cough: a randomized placebo controlled trial of treatment efficacy. *Thorax.* 2006;61: 1065-1069.
15. Maceri DR, Zim S. Laryngospasm: an atypical manifestation of severe gastroesophageal reflux disease (GERD). *Laryngoscope.* 2001;111(11):1976-1979.
16. Poelmans J, Tack J, Feenstra L. Paroxysmal laryngospasm: a typical but under recognized supraesophageal manifestation of gastroesophageal reflux? *Dig Dis Sci.* 2004;49(11-12),1868-1874.
17. Aviv JE, Liu H, Parides M, Kaplan ST, Close LG. Laryngopharyngeal sensory deficits in patients with laryngopharyngeal reflux and dysphagia. *Ann Otol Rhinol Laryngol.* 2000;109(11):1000-1006.
18. Thompson DM. Laryngopharyngeal sensory testing and assessment of airway protection in pediatric patients. *Am J Med.* 2003;18(115 suppl 3A):166S-168S.
19. Suskind DL, Thompson DM, Gulati M, Huddleston P, Liu DC, Baroody FM. Improved infant swallowing after gastroesophageal reflux disease treatment: a function of improved laryngeal sensation? *Laryngoscope.* 2006;116(8):1397-1403.
20. Jacobson BH, Johnson A, Grywalski C, Silbergleit A, Jacobson G, Benninger MS. The Voice Handicap Index (VHI): development and validation. *Am J Speech-Lang Path.* 1997;6(3):66-70.
21. Rosen CA, Lee AS, Osborne J, Zullo T, Murry T. Development and validation of the Voice Handicap Index-10. *Laryngoscope.* 2004;114(9):1549-1556.
22. Ma EP, Yiu EM. Voice activity and participation profile: assessing the impact of voice disorders on daily activities. *J Speech Lang Hear Res.* 2001;44(3):511-524.
23. Phua SY, McGarvey LP, Ngu MC, Ing AJ. Patients with gastro-esophageal reflux disease and cough have impaired laryngopharyngeal mechanosensitivity. *Thorax.* 2005;60(6):488-491.
24. Botoman VA. Noncardiac chest pain. *J Clin Gastroenterol.* 2002;34(1):6-14.
25. Hicks DM, Milstein CF. Laryngeal Hygiene. Merati AL, Bielamowicz SA, eds. In: *Textbook of Voice Disorders.* San Diego, Calif: Plural Publishing; 2007.
26. Murry T, Rosen CA. The role of the speech-language pathologist in the treatment of voice disorders. Rubin JS, Sataloff RT, Korovin GS, eds. In: *Diagnosis and Treatment of Voice Disorders*, 3rd ed. San Diego, Calif: Plural Publishing; 2006.
27. Altman KW, Atkinson C, Lazarus C. Current and emerging concepts in muscle tension dysphonia: a 30-month review. *J Voice.* 2005;19(2):261-267.
28. Christopher KL, Wood RP 2nd, Eckert RC, Blager FB, Raney RA, Souhrada JF. Vocal-cord dysfunction presenting as asthma. *N Engl J Med.* 1983;308(26):1566-1570.
29. Murry T, Tabaee A, Aviv JE. Respiratory retraining of refractory cough and laryngopharyngeal reflux in patients with paradoxical vocal fold movement disorder. *Laryngoscope.* 2004;114(8): 1341-1345.

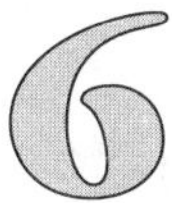

Globus

Ted Mau, Dale C. Ekbom, and
C. Gaelyn Garrett

Up to 46% of the population experience the sensation of a lump in the throat at one point or another.[1] Formerly considered an attribute of patients with hysteria, the condition was called *globus hystericus*. Remarkably, the term is still described in the psychiatric literature.[2] Today, globus is most commonly considered as an atypical symptom of GERD and a part of the symptom constellation associated with EER. In fact, globus is the number one symptom used anecdotally by otolaryngologists to diagnose reflux.[3,4] Consequently, patients who complain of globus are often assumed to have EER and started on antireflux therapy without consideration of other possible etiologies. However, GERD or EER are not the only disease entities that can give rise to globus. In this chapter, we review what is known about globus, conditions associated with globus, and recommendations for patient evaluation.

DEFINITION

The word *globus* comes from the Latin word for a ball. The globus symptom or globus sensation, the sensation of having a lump in the throat, has been described since the time of Hippocrates.[5] The condition was called *globus hystericus* because it was believed that the lump in the throat was caused by rising of the floating womb to the root of the neck in menopausal women, where it interfered with swallowing and sometimes breathing.[6] The condition was considered largely psychological and regarded as a sign of neurosis or hysteria. In 1794 the term "globus hystericus" was defined in the *Oxford English Dictionary* as "a choking sensation, as of a lump in the throat to which hysterical persons are subject."[7] It was not until the second half of the 20th century when physiologic causes for globus were seriously considered,[7] and the terms *globus pharyngeus*, *globus symptom*, and the more modern *globus sensation* came into use.

Patients almost never use the term "globus." Instead, they commonly describe a "lump" or "tightness" in the throat, a "choking" sensation, or "there is something in my throat that I feel I need to clear but can't bring up." This sensation is almost constant and is present outside of meal times. Patients do not report difficulty or pain with swallowing. In fact, the globus sensation tends to transiently abate during swallowing or is unchanged by it.

Even though the nature of the complaint is vague, the globus sensation can be defined as the persistent feeling of a lump, tightness, or choking sensation in the throat that has been present for weeks to months, independent of swallowing and in the absence of dysphagia. This should be distinguished from the transient sensation of throat tightness during times of acute stress.

CONDITIONS ASSOCIATED WITH GLOBUS

Association with Esophageal Dysmotility

Several studies in both the gastroenterology and otolaryngology literature have shown a high incidence of esophageal dysmotility in patients with globus. Over half of a group of globus patients were found to have achalasia or "hypochalasia."[8] Sixty-seven percent of another group of globus patients were found to have abnormal findings on manometry, with nonspecific esophageal motility disorder being the most frequent.[9] Seven of 12 globus patients in another study were also found to have nonspecific esophageal motility disorder.[10] It should be noted that none of these studies had an asymptomatic control group for comparison, and the relatively high incidence of esophageal dysmotility does not imply causation.

UES dysfunction was at one point postulated to be causative for the globus sensation, but evidence connecting the two is indirect, and negative evidence predominates. In Corso et al's retrospective review[11] of a cohort undergoing manometry, 62% of the patients who presented with globus had elevated resting UES tone, versus only 10% of those without globus. Earlier controlled studies did not find significant difference in the resting UES pressure between globus patients and controls.[12-14] In addition, in response to acute emotional stress[13] or esophageal distention,[15] globus patients demonstrated comparable increase in UES pressure versus controls but this did not elicit their symptom of globus. Corso et al[11] attributed the discrepancy between their study and the earlier ones to their use of more advanced manometric technology.

Wilson et al[14] showed some difference in pharyngoesophageal motility between globus patients and asymptomatic controls. In this prospective study, there was no significant difference between the groups in LES or resting UES pressures. However, globus patients showed significantly greater pharyngeal and UES after-contraction pressures and more complete UES relaxation than controls. The authors note that the latter observation may be an artifact due to greater catheter displacement during swallow in globus patients. They caution that although the differences in after-contraction pressures are real, it does not follow that they are clinically significant or are the cause of the globus sensation. Alternatively, the differences may contribute to the generation of the globus sensation, but possibly in association with other factors.

Although the literature does not provide strong evidence to link elevated resting UES tone with globus, it is generally accepted that UES spasm can cause globus, and that distal reflux events can trigger UES spasm. It is important to note that in this scenario, it is gastroesophageal reflux, rather than extraesophageal reflux, that is indirectly causing globus.

There is also some evidence that increased esophageal stretch may elicit the globus sensation. One study using esophageal balloon dilation in globus patients versus healthy controls showed the former to report globus sensation more frequently and at lower distention volumes than controls, suggesting that globus patients are more sensitive to esophageal stretch.[15] However, it should be noted that patients with complaints of globus have symptoms on a chronic basis, whereas in the experimental setting the globus sensation is elicited on a transient basis, and the two are probably not the same entity.

Association with GERD

Globus has long been associated with GERD and is considered an atypical symptom of GERD. However, evidence for esophageal reflux causing globus is indirect at best. In a generally healthy population interviewed, globus occurred in equal proportions in those with and without heartburn (43.5% vs 46.5%).[1] In a group of patients with EER symptoms who underwent EGD, globus was found in equal proportions in those with or without evidence of esophagitis (62% vs 71%).[16] Conversely, the incidence of heartburn was not found to be different between the general population and a cohort with globus (36% vs 38%).[17] Koufman found that almost half of the patients who complain of globus did not have heartburn or regurgitation.[18] These data are consistent with the notion that globus is attributable to one or more entities that are distinct from GERD.

Data from pH monitoring are also contradictory. The percentage of globus patients with abnormal distal reflux ranges from 23 to 65%.[14,18–21] Wilson et al[14] found the mean distal acid exposure time was not significantly different between globus patients and controls, and that only 23% of globus patients had elevated exposure times. In the same group of globus patients, only 18% had histologic esophagitis. In a review of all patients who underwent manometry at a single institution, 26% of globus patients had abnormal distal acid reflux, versus 39% of patients without globus.[11] Batch,[19] Timon et al,[20] and Koufman[18] reported 65%, 52%, and 50% of their globus patients, respectively, had abnormal distal acid reflux, but none of the studies had an asymptomatic control group. Timon et al[20] further reported that the presence or absence of heartburn had no bearing on treatment outcome. In a controlled study in a Chinese population with a low incidence of GERD, Hill et al[21] reported that 31% of globus patients had abnormal esophageal pH study, versus only 5% for non-globus controls. This was interpreted as supporting an association between GERD and globus. However, the control group all had prior normal EGD studies, and this inclusion criterion may have skewed the comparison. The authors concluded that despite the association, GERD is probably not causative in the majority of globus patients.

Although some of the discrepancy between the above studies may be due to different definitions of abnormal reflux, the evidence taken as a whole does not support a definitive link between abnormal distal reflux and globus.

Association with EER

The first inference that globus could be attributed to EER was made in 1970. Cherry et al[22] reported on a series of 12 patients with complaints ranging from "rawness or burning deep in the throat to a sensation of pressure or a lump in the throat." In some patients, this was also associated with mild hoarseness or paroxysmal cough. The symptoms were less severe during swallowing. Three of the 12 patients were shown to have frank esophagopharyngeal reflux on modified barium swallow, and 11 of the 12 patients demonstrated abnormal esophageal motility. All had marked improvement in their symptoms following strict dietary modification and intensive antacid regimen. The authors postulated that "pharyngeal localization" of reflux-induced symptoms could be mediated by reflex pathways triggered by distal esophageal reflux or by direct esophagopharyngeal reflux.

Globus is a prominent symptom among patients deemed to have laryngeal symptoms of reflux such as cough, throat clearing, and hoarseness. Percentage of these patients with globus as part of their symptom complex ranges from 12% to 67%.[10,16,18,23] Definitive evidence linking globus to abnormal hypopharyngeal acid reflux is lacking, however. In 18 patients with globus who underwent double-pH probe monitoring, only 28% had any pH drop below 4 in the hypopharynx during the 24-hour study period.[18] Another study, however, found 72% of globus patients with positive hypopharyngeal acid reflux by the same criteria.[24] Several studies examined symptom severity as relating to the presence of hypopharyngeal acid reflux in patients with EER symptoms. Two studies found that the severity of globus was the same between groups with or without hypopharyngeal acid reflux.[25,26] The interpretation of these data is controversial and is illustrative of the debate over how patients with EER symptoms should be managed.[27]

One growing area of investigation has to do with the role of nonacid reflux in causing EER symptoms. One study showed that for globus patients with persistent symptoms on BID PPI therapy, proximal reflux (as determined by impedance at 15 cm above the LES) was a significant predictor of globus symptom, and nonacid distal reflux approached significance in predicting globus.[28] Further studies looking at nonacid reflux will be important in clarifying the relationship between reflux and globus.

Association with Excessive Muscle Tension

Muscle tension dysphonia (MTD) is a common and probably underdiagnosed condition in patients presenting with laryngeal complaints. It was found in 38% of patients seen in a large referral voice center for the complaint of hoarseness,[29] and it is thought that up to 60 to 70% of patients in some voice clinics have MTD.[30] Patients with MTD often complain of hoarseness, vocal fatigue, and anterior neck pain or soreness with voice use. The associated throat tightness can also cause chronic cough and other laryngeal irritation symptoms. Anterior neck tenderness often can be reproduced by palpating the submental region or strap muscles at the thyrohyoid space. On laryngoscopic examination, supraglottic hyperfunction with anterior-posterior or lateral supraglottic squeeze (Color Plate 7) with glottal fry (inappropriate lower pitch with poor airflow) is characteristic.[31,32]

In contrast with the abundance of literature on reflux, few reports have examined the role of excessive muscle tension as an etiologic factor in patients with throat complaints typically considered EER symptoms. A retrospective review of 150 patients with a diagnosis of MTD showed globus as a symptom in only 5% of patients.[31] This is likely an underestimate if the patients were not specifically queried about globus during the visit. In our experience, some patients with MTD will also complain of a lump in the throat when specifically asked. We have a cohort of patients with voice complaints and MTD whose globus sensation is resolved after speech therapy. We suspect that the globus sensation in these patients may be the direct sensory correlate of excessive muscle tension, which in turn could be either primary in nature or secondary to underlying vocal fold pathology such as bowing or paresis.[32]

Association with Other Throat Complaints

Most studies examining the association between reflux and EER symptoms do not specify whether globus was the primary symptom, a secondary symptom, or the only symptom of the patients. In Koufman's landmark study of patients with EER symptoms, in the subgroup of patients with globus, the frequency of any other throat symptoms was about 50%.[18] In two large studies of globus patients, globus was the major or only symptom in 58% and 65% of the patients, respectively.[19,33] In another study of patients with globus as the primary symptom, 75% had associated throat symptoms such as throat clearing and dryness.[20] With a mean follow-up of 27 months, the authors found that patients *without* associated throat symptoms are more likely to respond to therapy, which consisted of antireflux measures for only those with esophagitis, and reassurance for those without. Almost half of the patients *with* associated throat symptoms did not improve with treatment. This implies that patients with associated symptoms may be less likely to have acid reflux as a cause of their symptoms. In contrast, Smit et al[34] found that patients with both globus and hoarseness are more likely to have abnormal distal esophageal acid reflux than patients with only globus or only hoarseness. The authors concluded that patients who complain of both symptoms should be worked up more aggressively. Most studies to date of patients with EER symptoms do not have the statistical power to perform subgroup analysis of patients with only one symptom. It may be useful to study patients who only complain of globus versus those who have other concomitant throat complaints to see if they have a different spectrum of etiologic factors.

Few reports contain data on the association of globus with vocal symptoms. Among a large group of patients with

EER symptoms, 50% of the subgroup with globus also complained of hoarseness.[18] In a study of patients with hoarseness, only 7% also complained of globus,[29] but this likely represents an underestimate as it was from self-reporting and not from active elicitation or a questionnaire.

Only one study to date examined the use of the Reflux Symptom Index (RSI) in globus patients. 77% of the globus patients had an RSI above 13.[24] Presumably the other 23% of patients had fewer and/or less severe other symptoms probed by the RSI. It is also a point of debate whether the RSI actually measures symptoms directly attributed to EER.[35]

Association with Psychological Conditions

Given its origin in antiquity, it is not surprising that globus is still associated with psychological conditions in modern times. Earlier studies suggested there was a high incidence of depression and obsessive traits in patients with globus, but few had true hysteria.[6,36] Later studies with control groups showed that female globus patients had significantly higher neuroticism scores than asymptomatic females,[37] and that psychological abnormalities are more common in patients with globus than in controls.[38] Other studies, however, did not find a difference.[8]

Psychological contribution to the globus symptom is often overlooked by throat specialists and those who treat reflux. Conversely, organic etiologies tend not to be the focus during evaluation of globus patients by psychiatrists. The literature reflects this specialty bias. Globus is considered a specific form of conversion disorder in the psychiatric literature.[2] A conversion disorder is defined by the presence of bodily symptoms judged to be due to psychological factors because the condition is preceded by conflicts or other stressors.[39] It should be obvious from the preceeding discussions that simple characterization of globus in the absence of physical abnormalities as a conversion disorder is probably imprudent.

While globus is probably not purely psychological in origin in many patients, the globus sensation is commonly seen in somatization disorder, where a patient has multiple somatic complaints in multiple organ systems that occur over several years in the absence of a medical condition. Approximately one-third of patients with this disorder report globus as a symptom.[40] Globus is reported to be the fourth most common symptom in these patients following vomiting, aphonia, and painful extremities.[41] Aside from the association with somatization disorder, a defined psychiatric illness, globus is also associated with somatization, the presentation of somatic symptoms in the absence of medical disease. Somatization often increases during periods of stress or conflict. Globus patients score high in the somatization dimension of a psychometrics questionnaire.[24] It has been reported that females with globus sensation are more often anxious, depressed, or show somatic concerns.[42]

Despite the data cited above, it should be emphasized that all these studies only report an association with globus and none has shown that treatment of the psychiatric condition relieves the globus sensation.

One study of globus patients that included both psychological testing and double-probe pH monitoring is of interest.[24] Globus patients with no hypopharyngeal acid reflux were found to have significantly higher psychological symptom scores than globus patients with hypopharyngeal acid reflux. This suggests that psychological factors play a major etiologic role in globus patients who do not have hypopharyngeal acid reflux. This finding has significant implication for the assessment and treatment of globus patients, as psychological evaluation is generally not part of the evaluation. It would be interesting to see how these two groups with demonstrated difference in psychological profile respond to a trial of PPIs.

It is possible that globus associated with psychological conditions is mediated through increased muscle tension. Many people have experienced the tightening of neck and shoulder musculature during times of stress, and it has been our observation that generalized tension in the neck and shoulder is often associated with tension in the extralaryngeal musculature. High psychological demand at work has been shown to be associated with pain in the neck and shoulders,[43] and workers with somatic symptoms are more likely to have neck discomfort.[44] The possibility of emotional stress as an indirect cause of globus in patients with high stress levels at home or work should be entertained.

In addition to being possibly causative for globus, psychological factors may interact with organic factors to perpetuate or enhance the globus sensation. In some patients, organic factors may initiate the symptom, which is then maintained by psychological factors such as operant conditioning.[45] In other patients, psychological factors such as emotional stress and anxiety may exacerbate globus that had an organic origin.[46] The interaction between psychological factors and globus has not been fully explored in the otolaryngology literature.

REVIEW OF CURRENT PRACTICE

Part of the controversy surrounding the diagnosis and treatment of EER suggested by patients with globus has to do with confusion of terminology. Patients with "EER symptoms," for example, globus, are often considered to in fact have EER before there is adequate workup. The use of empiric PPI administration in these patients is widely accepted as part of the workup, but many practitioners have come to regard the empiric administration as therapy and thus label patients with globus as having EER. A large survey showed that most otolaryngologists make the diagnosis of reflux more on symptoms than on laryngeal signs, and that globus and throat clearing were considered the most useful symptoms in diagnosing reflux.[3,4,47] However, these symptoms may represent the least specific markers for reflux. Symptoms commonly thought of as EER symptoms are symptoms of throat irritation and can be caused by a variety of factors including smoking, sinonasal drainage, voice abuse, or muscle tension. Current practice appears to over-emphasize the importance of reflux as the causative factor, with relatively little consideration to other possibilities. The overdiagnosis of reflux in the absence of adequate workup may be in large part due to the ease of prescribing PPIs as therapy, compared to the burden of additional referrals or workup. From a patient's perspective, it is also much easier to take a pill than to go for more appointments. However, much of the evidence, from individual studies[48–51] as well as meta-analyses,[52,53] suggests the therapeutic effects of PPIs are not significantly different from placebo.

It is also important to remember that globus, like other throat irritation symptoms, can be multifactorial in origin. EER, MTD, overuse/abuse/misuse of the voice, or other structural abnormalities of the laryngopharnx can occur simultaneously. Although some of these entities may be found at the same time, maybe only one or two directly contributes to globus sensation in a given patient, and a different factor in another patient with the same spectrum of findings may be causative in the other patient. To identify the etiologic factor(s) in any particular patient, skillful history taking is of the utmost importance.

HISTORY AND DIFFERENTIAL DIAGNOSES

Since patients almost never use the term "globus," it is important to not mislabel patients with globus when they, in fact, do not have globus. The duration of the symptom and variation of the symptom with swallowing should be carefully established. If the sensation of a lump in the throat is only present or is noticeably pronounced during swallowing, the possibility of a mass in the supraglottis or hypopharyx should be considered. If dysphagia is present, the patient likely does not have globus per se, and questioning should be directed toward symptoms of cricopharyngeal dysfunction, esophageal dysfunction, or mass effect. If the sensation of lump in the throat is transient and has only been present for a short time, it should not be considered typical globus. Patients with true globus usually have had the sensation for at least weeks to months, and the sensation persists for long periods of time, if not "all the time."

Patients should point to where the sensation is localized. The globus sensation is localized to the median or paramedian position in 75 to 80% of the patients, usually at the level of the cricoid or between the cricoid and the sternal notch.[14,19,20] If the sensation persistently localizes to one side and is very focal, an anatomic basis for the sensation should be suspected, for example, mass lesion, mucosal aberration, or focal sensory disturbance. A recent history of traumatic ingestion, for example, fishbone, should be elicited. If the sensation is localized to the back of the mouth, subsequent questioning and examination should be directed to the possibility of postnasal drip, mass in the oropharynx, or other sensory disturbance at the oropharynx level.

A history of unintentional weight loss associated with the sensation of a lump in the throat should alert the physician to explore other possibilities that could cause dysphagia or odynophagia. Typically a history of dysphagia or weight loss should direct the diagnostic process away from globus to something with a more defined anatomic basis, for example, esophageal dysmotility, pharyngeal pouch, or mass effect.

The onset of true globus is typically not discrete in time and not associated with particular events. If onset of symptom correlates with a particular event, it may give insight into the cause of the symptom. Was there a history of possible trauma, for example, intubation or foreign body ingestion? Was there nausea or vomiting? Did the globus sensation follow a choking episode? An antecedent such as choking or vomiting that was not excessive raises the possibility that globus could be the result of a positive feedback loop stemming from an unpleasant event associated with abnormal sensation of the throat.[46] This part of the history is important to elicit because it would point to psychological rather than organic modes of therapy.

Associated typical and atypical symptoms of reflux should be elicited. This part of history taking may be assisted by a questionnaire, so that every patient is asked the same set of symptoms, and no symptom is left out. It is also important to ask whether the associated symptoms occur at the same time as the globus sensation. For example, a patient with periods of throat clearing, chronic cough, and globus in which all three symptoms occur at the same time is more likely to have a "unifying diagnosis" such as EER or MTD than a patient whose cough tends to occur independently of globus. In the latter case, even though the patient complains of both cough and globus, the two may have different etiologies. If the patient has already been on a PPI, it is important to know how long they have been on the PPI, whether they have been taking it at the correct times, that is, before meals, and, most importantly, whether any symptoms changed with the use of PPI. It must be kept in mind that PPI administration in patients suspected of having EER is a diagnostic tool. A patient whose throat clearing, cough, and globus improve with PPI probably does have EER as the major culprit, even if there is coexisting MTD, for example. In our experience, patients whose globus symptom improves with PPI therapy tend to have typical GERD symptoms to begin with. The coexistence of typical GERD symptoms with globus during the initial encounter would place EER higher up on the diagnostic differential.

Symptoms consistent with excessive muscle tension should be explored. Is there any voice disturbance, vocal fatigue, or neck soreness with voice use? Does the sensation of lump in the throat correlate with prolonged voice use? Does the symptom persist during periods of rest and decreased voice use? Did the symptom start after a bout of URI? Frequently, patients complain of dysphonia that persists after other symptoms of URI have resolved, because they develop unfavorable compensatory phonatory techniques during the acute illness, and the resultant excessive tension becomes habitual during subsequent voice use. If the globus sensation began after URI and correlates with dysphonia, MTD as a cause of globus should be suspected.

While it is common to have the sensation of a lump in the throat during acute periods of emotional stress, the sensation should resolve when the stress trigger subsides. This transient response is not globus. However, as discussed above, globus can be associated with periods of prolonged or chronic psychological disturbance. Patients should be queried whether the symptom correlates with stressful periods at work or home, or whether the symptom was present during vacations or varied with significant changes in work cycle. Although it may not be prudent or acceptable to the patients to attribute their symptom solely to a psychiatric cause, it is reasonable to suggest, for patients who report correlation of symptom with stress, that it could be contributing to the sensation of globus. Patients who also have longstanding multiple vague complaints in multiple other organ systems should be suspected of having a somatization disorder and should be referred for psychiatric evaluation, if the physical examination is normal.

PHYSICAL EXAMINATION

Physical examination of the globus patient should encompass what is typically done for any patient with throat complaints referred to an otolaryngologist. The neck should be assessed for the presence of masses including goiter. Particular attention should then be paid to the presence or absence of excessive tightness in the extralaryngeal musculature. This consists of palpation of the submental space and the thyrohyoid space to assess the tension of the musculature at rest and during phonation. Palpation of the musculature spanning the thyrohyoid space is most diagnostic.[30] In a patient with globus along with dysphonia, the finding of excess muscle tension on examination suggests the possibility of MTD as a cause of both the dysphonia and globus.

Office visualization of the pharynx and larynx is mandatory for any globus patient to rule out structural abnormalities or masses. Hypertrophic tonsils can cause globus. Patients who have a supraglottic or hypopharyngeal mass or mucosal injury as the cause of globus are likely to also have dysphagia or odynophagia, which should have already been elicited from history taking and directed the physician's attention away from a case of typical globus. Nevertheless, it is certainly possible for an early tumor to present with globus, or for a small tumor in the petiole of the epiglottis or piriform sinus to be missed on office endoscopy. For this reason, the possibility of malignancy should always be kept in mind, and the appropriate workup or follow-up carried out based on other elements of the patient's history and physical examination.

DIAGNOSTIC TESTING

Most of the consideration of the "right" diagnostic testing for globus pertains to the larger question of what constitutes appropriate testing for patients with EER symptoms, an area of active controversy.[54,55] Few reports address diagnostic testing specific to globus. The roles of pH monitoring and upper GI endoscopy are discussed elsewhere in this text and are not explored here.

Barium swallow is not recommended for the purpose of excluding malignancy in patients with history consistent with true globus, that is, not associated with dysphagia, regurgitation, pain, or weight loss, and who do not have risk factors for malignancy and had normal office endoscopic laryngeal examination. Several retrospective reviews of large patient series who have undergone barium swallow found no cases of malignancy in this group of patients.[33,56,57] The most common findings from barium swallow were hiatal hernia and reflux. The few patients who did have significant findings, for example, malignancy, pharyngeal pouch or diverticulum, stricture, or web, all had symptoms in addition to globus. These findings would have been suspected based on history alone, and the barium swallow would have been ordered for a different indication. The authors commented that it is routine in some otolaryngology practices to order barium swallow as part of the workup for globus patients. Although it is more expedient than securing gastroenterology referral for possible endoscopy and/or pH monitoring, the diagnostic value does not justify the expense and unnecessary radiation exposure. A similar conclusion was reached regarding the diagnostic value of rigid endoscopy.[58]

Modified barium swallow (MBS), or videofluoroscopic swallow study, should be obtained for patients whose history is consistent with dysphagia and/or aspiration. The use of MBS to assess globus in the absence of dysphagia is likely to have a low diagnostic yield, as most conditions associated with globus as reviewed above are not adequately assessed with MBS. A few reports in the literature do not suggest definitive guidelines. A case-control study of globus patients versus dysphagia patients showed 16% of globus patients with early closure of the cricopharyngeus compared to 2% of dysphagia patients.[59] A prospective study of globus patients showed one-third with abnormal findings, including aspiration, stasis of barium in the vallecula and piriform sinuses, and poor laryngeal elevation.[60] Whether these findings are clinically significant or causative is unclear. A large retrospective study found significant incidence of abnormalities on MBS for globus patients who did not complain of dysphagia.[61] The most frequent abnormalities found were nonspecific esophageal motor disorders, pharyngoesophageal sphincter dysfunction, and pharyngeal stasis. The dilemma in interpreting these results revolves around whether these findings are relevant, and if so, in which patients and what to do about them.

In-office transnasal esophagoscopy (TNE) has been advocated as a screening examination for patients with reflux, globus, or dysphagia.[62] In the largest series reported, approximately 1 out of 6 patients examined had findings of esophagitis, 7% had a hiatal hernia, and 5% had Barrett's metaplasia.[62] These and other findings of lower frequency were taken as evidence to support the use of TNE. The same authors later reported that only 30% of the patients with endoscopic evidence of Barrett's had biopsy-proven Barrett's metaplasia.[63] Another report found the prevalence of esophagitis and Barrett's metaplasia to be less than 20% in patients with pH-documented laryngopharyngeal reflux.[64] No data have been reported specifically on globus patients. Most of the evidence supporting the utility of TNE has come from a few select centers. Broader, independent validation would be useful in elucidating the diagnostic value of TNE in globus patients.

MANAGEMENT

The management of the globus patient is not monolithic. For any given individual, the strategy depends on the index of suspicion for specific etiologic factors. This index of suspicion is largely derived from the history, with contributions from examination findings. Selected scenarios illustrate this approach. If reflux is suspected, the options include pH monitoring with or without manometry, an empiric trial of PPIs, or in-office transnasal esophagoscopy. If the history suggests globus along with MTD, the examination shows laryngeal hyperfunction, and the patient is also dysphonic, a trial of voice therapy may be useful (Fig 6–1). It is important for the physician to follow up with the patient after voice therapy to inquire whether the globus sensation has diminished. Some patients may have reflux coexisting with MTD, and the globus may be due to one or the other or both. This should be discussed with the

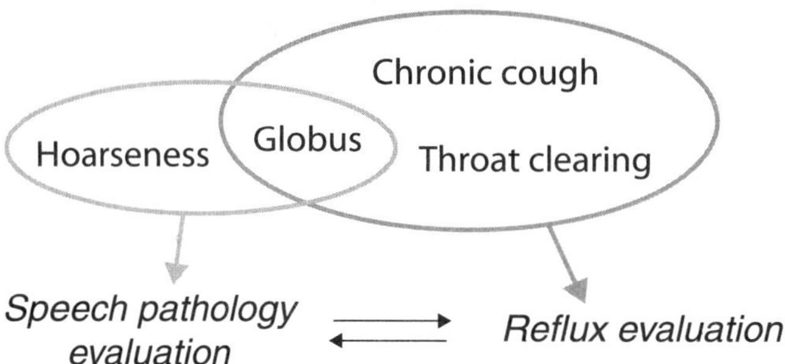

Fig 6–1. For a given patient, associated laryngeal irritation symptoms in addition to globus can help direct the choice of initial evaluation. For example, a patient with globus and hoarseness with evidence of excessive muscle tension on exam may benefit from speech therapy evaluation initially. A patient with globus, throat clearing, chronic cough, and signs of LPR may benefit from initial evaluation for reflux.

patient. Workup and/or trial therapy for one or both possible etiologic factors can be initiated. If the suspicion for reflux is low, the examination is normal, and the patient gives history of multiple psychological stressors, consideration can be given for reassurance and suitable followup.

CONCLUSION

Globus has different etiologic factors in different patients, and it may be multifactorial in any given patient. To make the correct diagnosis requires an understanding of the various causes of globus and broad thinking to include all of them in history taking. These may include reflux, esophageal pathology, excessive muscle tension, or psychological factors. The use of PPIs may be useful in select patients as a diagnostic tool, but follow-up is required and the medication should be discontinued if the patients do not respond. As with the entire field of EER, further studies are necessary to provide more science and clarity to the management of the globus patient.

REFERENCES

1. Thompson WG, Heaton KW. Heartburn and globus in apparently healthy people. *Can Med Assoc J.* 1982;126:46–48.
2. Finkenbine R, Miele VJ. Globus hystericus: a brief review. *Gen Hosp Psychiatry.* 2004;26:78–82.
3. Ahmed TF, Khandwala F, Abelson TI, et al. Chronic laryngitis associated with gastroesophageal reflux: prospective assessment of differences in practice patterns between gastroenterologists and ENT physicians. *Am J Gastroenterol.* 2006;101:470–478.
4. Karkos PD, Benton J, Leong SC, et al. Trends in laryngopharyngeal reflux: a British ENT survey. *Eur Arch Otorhinolaryngol.* 2007;264:513–517.

5. Adams F. *The Genuine Works of Hippocrates.* London: The Syndenham Society; 1894.
6. Pratt LW, Tobin WH, Gallagher RA. Globus hystericus—office evaluation by phychological testing with the MMPI. *Laryngoscope.* 1976;86:1540-1551.
7. Malcomson KG. Globus hystericus vel pharyngis. *J Laryngol Otol.* 1968;82: 219-230.
8. Moser G, Vacariu-Granser GV, Schneider C, et al. High incidence of esophageal motor disorders in consecutive patients with globus sensation. *Gastroenterology.* 1991;101:1512-1521.
9. Farkkila MA, Ertama L, Katila H, et al. Globus pharyngis, commonly associated with esophageal motility disorders. *Am J Gastroenterol.* 1994;89:503-508.
10. Knight RE, Wells JR, Parrish RS. Esophageal dysmotility as an important co-factor in extraesophageal manifestations of gastroesophageal reflux. *Laryngoscope.* 2000;110:1462-1466.
11. Corso MJ, Pursnani KG, Mohiuddin MA, et al. Globus sensation is associated with hypertensive upper esophageal sphincter but not with gastroesophageal reflux. *Dig Dis Sci.* 1998;43:1513-1517.
12. Caldarelli DD, Andrews AH Jr, Derbyshire AJ. Esophageal motility studies in globus sensation. *Ann Otol Rhinol Laryngol.* 1970;79(6):1098-1100.
13. Cook IJ, Dent J, Collins SM. Upper esophageal sphincter tone and reactivity to stress in patients with a history of globus sensation. *Dig Dis Sci.* 1989;34: 672-676.
14. Wilson JA, Pryde A, Piris J, et al. Pharyngoesophageal dysmotility in globus sensation. *Arch Otolaryngol Head Neck Surg.* 1989;115:1086-1090.
15. Cook IJ, Shaker R, Dodds WJ, Hogan WJ, Arndorfer RC. Role of mechanical and chemical stimulation of the esophagus in globus sensation. *Gastroenterology.* 1989;96:A99.
16. Tauber S, Gross M, Issing WJ. Association of laryngopharyngeal symptoms with gastroesophageal reflux disease. *Laryngoscope.* 2002;112:879-886.
17. Moloy PJ, Charter R. The globus symptom. Incidence, therapeutic response, and age and sex relationships. *Arch Otolaryngol.* 1982;108:740-744.
18. Koufman JA. The otolaryngologic manifestations of gastroesophageal reflux disease (GERD): a clinical investigation of 225 patients using ambulatory 24-hour pH monitoring and an experimental investigation of the role of acid and pepsin in the development of laryngeal injury. *Laryngoscope.* 1991;101(4 pt 2, suppl 53):1-78.
19. Batch AJ. Globus pharyngeus (Pt I). *J Laryngol Otol.* 1988;102:152-158.
20. Timon C, O'Dwyer T, Cagney D, Walsh M. Globus pharyngeus: long-term follow-up and prognostic factors. *Ann Otol Rhinol Laryngol.* 1991;100:351-354.
21. Hill J, Stuart RC, Fung HK, et al. Gastroesophageal reflux, motility disorders, and psychological profiles in the etiology of globus pharyngis. *Laryngoscope.* 1997; 107:1373-1377.
22. Cherry J, Siegel CI, Margulies SI, Donner M. Pharyngeal localization of symptoms of gastroesophageal reflux. *Ann Otol Rhinol Laryngol.* 1970;79:912-914.
23. Jacob P, Kahrilas PJ, Herzon G. Proximal esophageal pH-metry in patients with "reflux laryngitis." *Gastroenterology.* 1991;100:305-310.
24. Park KH, Choi SM, Kwon SU, Yoon SW, Kim SU. Diagnosis of laryngopharyngeal reflux among globus patients. *Otolaryngol Head Neck Surg.* 2006;134:81-85.
25. Noordzij JP, Khidr A, Desper E, et al. Correlation of pH probe-measured laryngopharyngeal reflux with symptoms and signs of reflux laryngitis. *Laryngoscope.* 2002;112:2192-2195.
26. Eubanks TR, Omelanczuk PE, Maronian N, et al. Pharyngeal pH monitoring in 222 patients with suspected laryngeal reflux. *J Gastrointest Surg.* 2001;5:183-190.
27. Vaezi MF, Hicks DM, Abelson TI, Richter JE. Laryngeal signs and symptoms and

gastroesophageal reflux disease (GERD): a critical assessment of cause and effect association. *Clin Gastroenterol Hepatol.* 2003;1:333-344.
28. Anandasabapathy S, Jaffin BW. Multichannel intraluminal impedance in the evaluation of patients with persistent globus on proton pump inhibitor therapy. *Ann Otol Rhinol Laryngol.* 2006;115:563-570.
29. Cohen SM, Garrett CG. Hoarseness: is it really laryngopharyngeal reflux? *Laryngoscope.* 2008;118(2):363-366.
30. Angsuwarangsee T, Morrison M. Extrinsic laryngeal muscular tension in patients with voice disorders. *J Voice.* 2002;16:333-343.
31. Altman KW, Atkinson C, Lazarus C. Current and emerging concepts in muscle tension dysphonia: a 30-month review. *J Voice.* 2005;19:261-267.
32. Belafsky PC, Postma GN, Reulbach TR, Holland BW, Koufman JA. Muscle tension dysphonia as a sign of underlying glottal insufficiency. *Otolaryngol Head Neck Surg.* 2002;127:448-451.
33. Back GW, Leong P, Kumar R, Corbridge R. Value of barium swallow in investigation of globus pharyngeus. *J Laryngol Otol.* 2000;114:951-954.
34. Smit CF, van Leeuwen JA, Mathus-Vliegen LM, et al. Gastropharyngeal and gastroesophageal reflux in globus and hoarseness. *Arch Otolaryngol Head Neck Surg.* 2000;126:827-830.
35. Wootten CT, Lutfi RE, Courey MS, Garrett CG. Discordance between clinical signs and ambulatory pH-probe monitoring in the diagnosis of laryngopharyngeal reflux. *Trans Amer Laryngol Assoc.* 2005;126:30.
36. Puhakka H, Lehtinen V, Aalto T. Globus hystericus—a psychosomatic disease? *J Laryngol Otol.* 1976;90:1021-1026.
37. Wilson JA, Deary IJ, Maran AG. Is globus hystericus? *Br J Psychiatry.* 1988;153:335-339.
38. Clouse RE. Psychiatric disorders in patients with esophageal disease. *Med Clin North Am.* 1991;75:1081-1096.
39. Sadock BJ, Sadock VA. *Kaplan and Sadock's Comprehensive Textbook of Psychiatry*, 8th ed. Philadelphia, Pa: Lippincott Williams & Wilkins; 2005.
40. Perley MJ, Guze SB. Hysteria—the stability and usefulness of clinical criteria. *N Engl J Med.* 1962;266:421-426.
41. Othmer E, DeSousa C. A screening test for somatization disorder (hysteria). *Am J Psychiatry.* 1985;142:1146-1149.
42. Deary IJ, Wilson JA, Mitchell L, et al. Covert psychiatric disturbances in patients with globus pharyngitis. *Br J Med Psychol.* 1989;62:381-389.
43. Leroyer A, Edme JL, Vaxevanoglou X, et al. Neck, shoulder, and hand and wrist pain among administrative employees: relation to work-time organization and psychosocial factors at work. *J Occup Environ Med.* 2006;48:326-333.
44. Pietri-Taleb F, Riihimaki H, Viikari-Juntura E, Lindstrom K. Longitudinal study on the role of personality characteristics and psychological distress in neck trouble among working men. *Pain.* 1994;58:261-267.
45. Solyom L, Sookman D. Fear of choking and its treatment. A behavioural approach. *Can J Psychiatry.* 1980;25:30-34.
46. Bishop LC, Riley WT. The psychiatric management of the globus syndrome. *Gen Hosp Psychiatry.* 1988;10:214-219.
47. Book DT, Rhee JS, Toohill RJ, Smith TL. Perspectives in laryngopharyngeal reflux: an international survey. *Laryngoscope.* 2002;112:1399-1406.
48. Noordzij JP, Khidr A, Evans BA, et al. Evaluation of omeprazole in the treatment of reflux laryngitis: a prospective, placebo-controlled, randomized, double-blind study. *Laryngoscope.* 2001;111:2147-2151.
49. Steward DL, Wilson KM, Kelly DH, et al. Proton pump inhibitor therapy for chronic laryngo-pharyngitis: a randomized placebo-control trial. *Otolaryngol Head Neck Surg.* 2004;131:342-350.
50. Eherer AJ, Habermann W, Hammer HF, et al. Effect of pantoprazole on the course of reflux-associated laryngitis: a placebo-

controlled double-blind crossover study. *Scand J Gastroenterol.* 2003;38:462-467.

51. Vaezi MF, Richter JE, Stasney CR, et al. Treatment of chronic posterior laryngitis with esomeprazole. *Laryngoscope.* 2006; 116:254-260.
52. Qadeer MA, Phillips CO, Lopez AR, et al. Proton pump inhibitor therapy for suspected GERD-related chronic laryngitis: a meta-analysis of randomized controlled trials. *Am J Gastroenterol.* 2006;101: 2646-2654.
53. Gatta L, Vaira D, Sorrenti G, et al. Meta-analysis: the efficacy of proton pump inhibitors for laryngeal symptoms attributed to gastro-oesophageal reflux disease. *Aliment Pharmacol Ther.* 2007;25: 385-392.
54. Belafsky PC. PRO: Empiric treatment with PPIs is not appropriate without testing. *Am J Gastroenterol.* 2006;101:6-8.
55. Vaezi MF. CON: treatment with PPIs should not be preceded by pH monitoring in patients suspected of laryngeal reflux. *Am J Gastroenterol.* 2006;101:8-10.
56. Harar RP, Kumar S, Saeed MA, Gatland DJ. Management of globus pharyngeus: review of 699 cases. *J Laryngol Otol.* 2004;118:522-527.
57. Hajioff D, Lowe D. The diagnostic value of barium swallow in globus syndrome. *Int J Clin Pract.* 2004;58:86-89.
58. Takwoingi YM, Kale US, Morgan DW. Rigid endoscopy in globus pharyngeus: how valuable is it? *J Laryngol Otol.* 2006;120:42-46.
59. Chung JY, Levine MS, Weinstein GS, Laufer I. Globus sensation: findings on videofluoroscopic examinations. *Can Assoc Radiol J.* 2003;54:35-40.
60. Chen CL, Tsai CC, Chou AS, Chiou JH. Utility of ambulatory pH monitoring and videofluoroscopy for the evaluation of patients with globus pharyngeus. *Dysphagia.* 2007;22:16-19.
61. Schima W, Pokieser P, Schober E, et al. Globus sensation: value of static radiography combined with videofluoroscopy of the pharynx and oesophagus. *Clin Radiol.* 1996;51:177-185.
62. Postma GN, Cohen JT, Belafsky PC, et al. Transnasal esophagoscopy: revisited (over 700 consecutive cases). *Laryngoscope.* 2005;115:321-323.
63. Halum SL, Postma GN, Bates DD, Koufman JA. Incongruence between histologic and endoscopic diagnoses of Barrett's esophagus using transnasal esophagoscopy. *Laryngoscope.* 2006;116:303-306.
64. Koufman JA, Belafsky PC, Bach KK, Daniel E, Postma GN. Prevalence of esophagitis in patients with pH-documented laryngopharyngeal reflux. *Laryngoscope.* 2002;112:1606-1609.

7

Asthma and GER

Susan M. Harding

INTRODUCTION

Asthma is a heterogeneous disease with multiple distinct phenotypes in which many triggers and or contributing comorbid conditions lead to bronchospasm and lung inflammation.[1] Gastroesophageal reflux (GER) is a potential trigger or contributing factor of asthma.[2] Asthma and GER are both common diseases in our population and may coexist without a direct interaction.[3] Asthma afflicts 20 million persons in the United States with an adult prevalence rate of 6.7% and it is more prevalent in females (8.1%) compared to males (6.2%).[4] In 2003, asthma resulted in 12.3 million physician office visits, 1.8 million emergency department visits, 504,000 asthma hospital discharges, and 4210 deaths.[4] Controlling potential asthma triggers, such as GER, may improve asthma outcomes.

The relationship between asthma and GER remains controversial although evidence documents a clear interaction between the two disease states. Causality cannot be proven presently. To solidify the association between asthma and GER, three criteria should be considered: (1) Asthmatics should have a higher GER incidence or prevalence than individuals without asthma; (2) Pathophysiologic mechanisms should explain how the two disease processes interact; and (3) More convincingly, if GER triggers asthma, then GER therapy should improve asthma outcomes.[5] This chapter reviews the epidemiology of GER in asthmatics, examines predisposing factors for GER development in asthmatics, and examines mechanisms of GER-induced lung responses, and asthma outcomes with GER therapy. Finally, diagnostic and management strategies for GER in asthmatics along with current controversies are reviewed.

GER EPIDEMIOLOGY IN ASTHMATICS

Multiple population-based studies note an association between asthma and GER. A case-controlled study involving 101,366 veterans discharged from 172 Veterans Administration Hospitals noted that veterans with esophageal disease were more likely to have asthma than veterans without esophageal disease (odds ratio [*OR*] 1.15, 95% confidence interval [95% *CI*], 1.43–1.59).[6] Hancox and colleagues noted an association between respiratory symptoms, lung function, and GER symptoms in a population-based birth cohort of more than 1000 individuals.[7] Heartburn and regurgitation were significantly associated with asthma (*OR* 3.2, 95% *CI*, 1.6–6.4), wheezing (*OR* 3.5, 95% *CI*, 1.7–7.2), and nocturnal cough (*OR* 4.3, 95% *CI*, 2.1–8.7). In a cohort of more than 65,000 individuals representing 71% of the adult population in a Norwegian county, 5.4% had severe GER symptoms.[8] Asthmatics had GER to a 60% greater extent than individuals without asthma. Furthermore, there was a dose-response noted between breathlessness and GER symptoms.[8] These population-based studies confirm that asthma and GER can interact.

There also are data examining the incidence of GER and asthma over a mean follow up period of three years in more than 15,000 patients having a first diagnosis of asthma or GER, and in more than 17,000 matched controls.[9] Patients with a first diagnosis of asthma had a significant increased risk of subsequent GER development, even when controlling for confounding factors.

Esophageal symptoms are also more prevalent in asthmatics compared to controls. Field et al[10] examined 109 asthmatics and 135 subjects in two control groups, finding that heartburn was present in 77% of asthmatics, compared to 52% and 48% of subjects in the two control groups (p <.05). The week before completing the questionnaire, 41% of the asthmatics had reflux-associated respiratory symptoms, and 28% used their inhaler while experiencing GER symptoms.[10] This questionnaire-based cross-sectional study shows that asthmatics associated their GER symptoms with their asthma symptoms. Selecting every 14th patient in a cohort of 2,225 asthmatics, Kiljander and colleagues noted that 52% had GER symptoms.[11]

Esophageal dysmotility, including lower esophageal sphincter (LES) hypotension and esophagitis is also prevalent in asthmatics. Kjellen et al[12] found that 38% of 97 consecutive asthmatics had esophageal dysmotility and 27% had LES hypotension. Sontag et al[13] noted that compared to controls, asthmatics had significantly lower LES pressures. Esophagitis prevalence was 43% in 186 consecutive asthmatics.[14]

Sontag et al[13] also noted that esophageal acid contact times are higher in asthmatics compared to control subjects. Eighty-two percent of consecutive asthmatics had abnormal esophageal acid contact times.

There was also a temporal correlation noted between respiratory symptoms and esophageal acid events, where 78% of respiratory symptoms were associated with esophageal acid events in asthmatics.[15] Not all asthmatics with significant GER have esophageal GER symptoms. In consecutive asthmatics without typical GER symptoms, 62% had abnormal esophageal acid contact times consistent with GER.[16] Table 7–1 reviews important prevalence information.

Gastroesophageal reflux is also a risk factor for frequent exacerbations in difficult-to-control asthma with an odds ratio of 4.9.[17] Similarly, in 42 consecutive difficult-to-control asthmatics, GER was a significant contributing factor.[18] Treatment of GER improved asthma outcomes in these difficult to control asthmatics.[18]

Although large population-based studies have the potential to include biases,

Table 7–1. GER Epidemiology and Prevalence in Asthmatics

• Increased GER prevalence and incidence in asthmatics
• GER symptoms—51 to 77%
• GER-associated asthma symtoms—41%
• Esophageal dysmotility—38%
• Lower esophageal sphincter pressure hypotension—27%
• Esophagitis—43%
• Abnormal esophageal acid contact times—82%
• GER symptom correlation with asthma symptoms—78%

evidence supports that GER prevalence is higher in asthmatics compared to the general population. That esophageal acid is temporally associated with respiratory symptoms further supports that esophageal acid can potentially trigger an asthma-type response.

FACTORS PROMOTING GER IN ASTHMA

There are many potential factors that may promote GER in asthmatics as primarily noted in observational studies. Potential factors include autonomic dysregulation, an increased pressure gradient between the thorax and the abdominal cavity, crural diaphragm dysfunction, and the use of asthma medications.[19] Asthmatics with GER have evidence of autonomic dysregulation with a hypervagal response or a mixed hypervagal hyperadrenergic response noted in 65%.[20] Autonomic dysregulation could impact LES pressure generation and frequency of transient relaxations of the LES. Furthermore, there is a potential increase in the pressure gradient between the thorax and abdominal cavity. At end expiration, the pressure gradient between the stomach and the esophagus approximates 5 mm Hg.[21] Thus, a normal LES pressure at end expiration is sufficient to counteract this pressure gradient.[21] However, if airflow obstruction is present, as in an asthma exacerbation, this pressure gradient may be surpassed, thus promoting GER.[21] The crural diaphragm contributes to LES pressure generation and hyperinflation associated with bronchospasm can place the crural diaphragm at a functional disadvantage because of geometric flattening.[21,22] Furthermore, asthma medications can impact GER. Theophylline increases esophageal acid contact times and decreases LES pressure.[23] Oral and inhaled beta-2 adrenergic agonists alter esophageal motility.[24,25] Oral corticosteroids increased esophageal acid contact times in one placebo-controlled trial.[26] Obesity may also predispose to GER in asthmatics.[27] All of these factors could potentially explain the increased GER prevalence in asthmatics.

GER-INDUCED LUNG RESPONSES

There are many potential mechanisms by which esophageal contents can induce bronchoconstriction, impact airway inflammation, and increase minute ventilation. Potential mechanisms include a vagal-esophageal-bronchial reflex, active local axonal reflexes, heightened bronchial reactivity, and microaspiration of esophageal contents into the upper airway.[19]

The lung and the esophagus share common embryonic foregut origins and autonomic innervation through the vagus nerve.[19] In animals models, acid in the esophagus is associated with an increase in respiratory resistance that is ablated with bilateral vagotomy.[28] In humans, esophageal acid increases airway resistance and reduces airflow and arterial oxygen saturation.[29,30] Atropine pretreatment abolishes these findings.[30] Our laboratory showed that microaspiration was not required to elicit bronchoconstriction, and vagolytic doses of atropine partially ablated this response, favoring a vagally-mediated reflex mechanism.[31-33] This vagal mechanism is further supported by an investigation showing that asthmatics with GER have autonomic dysregulation with a hypervagal state.[20]

In addition to a vagally-mediated reflex, local axonal reflexes may impact lung responses so that the central nervous system is not required. In guinea pigs, a neuronal connection exists between the esophagus and the lung with nitric oxide-containing neurons, and esophageal acid causes marked airway edema.[34] Tachykinin receptor antagonists prevents this airway response—verifying that nonvagal peripheral pathways acting through the autonomic ganglia may also be active.[35] Also, in these experiments the upper esophagus was ligated to prevent microaspiration.[35]

Esophageal reflux may also enhance bronchial reactivity. In 105 consecutive asthmatics, the degree of methacholine reactivity correlated with episodes of acid reflux during 24-hour esophageal pH monitoring.[36] Esophageal acid also impacts voluntary isocapnic hyperventilation of dry air and methacholine inhalation challenges tests. In asthmatics, the dose of methacholine required to produce a 20% fall in FEV_1 (PD_{20}) was significantly reduced during esophageal acid infusion compared with saline solution.[37] Vagal pathways are also important in this mechanism as this bronchial response was abolished with atropine pretreatment.[37] In 29 asthmatics, omeprazole 20 mg twice daily decreased the tussive response to capsaicin in asthmatics with GER which correlated with proximal acid exposure.[38] Thus, esophageal acid can alter bronchial airway responsiveness to methacholine as well as the tussive response to capsaicin.[38] Esophageal acid can also heighten bronchial reactivity during sleep. Acid reflux episodes correlated with increases in lower airway resistance in 7 asthmatics with GER.[39]

Microaspiration of esophageal contents into the airway can also elicit airway responses. In a cat model, 10 mL of esophageal acid caused a 1.5-fold increase in total lung resistance, compared to a 5-fold increase when 50 μL was instilled into the trachea.[40] In this microaspiration model, cervical vagotomy ablated the respiratory effects.[40] In a dog model, laryngeal instillation of acid and pepsin impaired important airway patency maintaining mechanisms, predisposing to laryngeal penetration and further episodes of microaspiration.[41] Microaspiration can also impact airway responses in humans. Monitoring tracheal and esophageal pH simultaneously in asthmatics with GER, esophageal acid decreased peak expiratory flow rate (PEF) 8 L/min.[42] Conversely, if microaspiration occurred, as documented by a fall in tracheal pH, PEF decreased 84 L/min.[42] Episodes of tracheal microaspiration were associated with more significant deterioration in airflow compared to episodes when esophageal acid alone was present.

Other studies, however, have failed to show significant airway responses with esophageal acid.[43] In a review of 14 investigations, Field and colleagues[44] noted that esophageal acid did cause airway responses, although they were minimal. This group went on to explore other factors that could explain the respiratory symptoms associated with GER. They noted in normal control subjects that esophageal acid was associated with increases in minute ventilation and respiratory rates that decreased with esophageal acid clearance.[45] These findings may explain the paradox of how GER can worsen respiratory symptoms without necessarily altering pulmonary airflow significantly. This study needs to be repeated in asthmatics. Of note, asthma is a highly heterogeneous disease, so bronchoconstrictor responses to esophageal acid may not be present in all asthmatics with GER but only those with GER-triggered asthma.

Asthma is an inflammatory disease, so if GER is a trigger of asthma, GER should lead to airway inflammation. In an animal model, esophageal acid caused the release of substance P which was associated with airway edema.[35] Tachykinins, including substance P and neurokinins, contract airway smooth muscle, increase bronchial mucous gland secretion, and increase vascular permeability.[35] In a guinea pig model, inhaled citric acid caused a dose-dependent increase in total pulmonary resistance, mediated by activation of sensory nerves and the release of tachykinins from peripheral nerve terminals.[46] This bronchoconstriction effect was reversed by pretreatment with a tachykinin NK-1 receptor antagonist.[46]

Evidence of tachykinin release is also noted in asthmatics with GER. Substance P and neurokinin A levels in induced sputum were significantly higher in asthmatics with acid GER as documented by esophageal pH testing compared to asthmatics without acid GER.[47] These data support the theory that sensory nerve activation is present in the airways of a subgroup of asthmatics.[47] Nitric oxide is another biomarker. In asthmatic children, exhaled nitric oxide levels were lower in asthmatic children with GER compared with asthmatic children without GER.[48] Nitric oxide results in bronchodilatation.[48] Asthmatics with GER also had evidence of eosinophilic inflammation and increased concentrations of interleukin-4 noted in exhaled breath condensates and induced sputum samples.[49] Furthermore, asthmatics with GER had evidence of oxidative stress as noted by a concomitant increase in 8-isoprostane concentration.[50] Two months of treatment with the proton-pump inhibitor (PPI) lansoprazole 30 mg/day lowered the 8-isoprostane concentration significantly.[50] This reduction in 8-isoprostane concentration in exhaled breath condensate was not noted in asthmatics without GER.[50]

Esophageal GER contents other than acid may also impact inflammatory mediators. Esophageal fluid osmolality can initiate local axonal reflexes and esophageal distention alone can initiate vagal reflexes. Airway epithelial cells can also release growth factors that promote fibroblastic proliferation.[51] The bile acid content in induced sputums of asthmatics with GER-associated symptoms was higher than in healthy control subjects.[52] These findings were associated with an increase in TGF-beta-1 messenger RNA expression.[52] These findings show that microaspiration of bile acid may induce airway fibrosis through the production of TGF-beta-1 and fibroblastic proliferation.

In conclusion, there are multiple potential pathophysiologic mechanisms whereby esophageal contents can induce bronchoconstriction and increase minute ventilation. Data from both animal and human investigations continue to support the hypothesis that esophageal contents can: (1) induce neurogenic and eosinophilic inflammation, (2) alter markers of oxidative stress, and (3) potentially induce a fibroblastic response in the airways.

ASTHMA OUTCOMES WITH GER THERAPY

If GER triggers asthma, then aggressive GER therapy should improve asthma outcomes in selected asthmatics. As an individual asthmatic may have multiple triggers, elimination of one trigger may not impact asthma outcomes. There are no diagnostic tests available to determine whether an individual asthmatic has GER-triggered asthma.[3] Multiple studies have examined asthma outcomes with GER therapy. Many of them have design flaws, including lack of a placebo arm, crossover design if a placebo arm is present, small subject populations, inadequate treatment duration, and inadequate evaluation of asthma and GER outcomes.[3] Two analyses published in 1998 and 2001 showed that there was objective improvement in asthma symptoms with minimal improvement in pulmonary function with GER therapy.[53,54] A recent Cochrane Database review concluded that GER therapy resulted in no consistent benefit for asthmatics.[55] Harding et al[56] noted that asthmatics often required aggressive acid suppression with twice-daily PPI use with a treatment duration of at least 12 weeks for improvement in asthma outcomes. Since 2000, five randomized placebo-controlled trials, which were not crossover in design, utilizing adequate amounts of a PPI for a minimum duration of 12 weeks, were performed in carefully defined asthmatics.[57-61] Two of these trials also evaluated subjects with esophageal pH testing and carefully evaluated GER variables prior to randomization.[60,61] Compiling the results from these 5 trials show that in 1,205 subjects, asthma symptoms and quality of life improved in the majority of treated subjects.[57-61] Some investigations showed improvement in PEF, especially in selected asthmatics.[59,61] Only one trial performed by Sharma et al[61] utilizing a PPI with a prokinetic agent noted improvement in PEF, FEV_1, and FVC. Table 7-2 reviews these double-blind randomized placebo-controlled trials using PPIs for an adequate duration and in a noncrossover manner.[57-61]

Kiljander et al[59] evaluated asthmatics with and without GER symptoms using esomeprazole 40 mg twice daily, for 16 weeks in one of these trials. Subjects with GER symptoms and nocturnal asthma symptoms had significant improvements in morning and evening PEF compared with the placebo group.[59] Furthermore, in a post hoc analysis, subjects on long-acting beta-agonists (LABAs) had more pronounced results.[59] Asthmatics who did not have GER or nocturnal asthma symptoms had no improvement in PEF with GER therapy. In another trial, Littner and coworkers[58] noted that PPI therapy resulted in improved quality of life and fewer asthma exacerbations. In a post hoc analysis, asthmatics receiving one or more asthma control medications, in addition to inhaled corticosteroids, were more likely to improve.[58] Both of these investigations note that selected

Table 7–2. Double-Blind, Randomized, Placebo-Controlled (Non-Crossover) Trials Utilizing Proton-Pump Inhibitors

Reference	Subjects	Medication	Duration	Outcome
Boeree MI et al.[57] *Eur Resp J.* 1998;111:1070	36 Single-site	Omeprazole 40 mg twice daily	12 wks	Improved nocturnal cough; no change in PFTs
Littner MR et al.[58] *Chest.* 2005;128:1128	207 Multi-center	Lansoprazole 30 mg twice daily	24 wks	Decreased asthma exacerbations, improved QOL; no improvement in asthma symptoms, PFT, or albuterol use
Kiljander TO et al.[59] *Am J Respir Crit Care Med.* 2006; 173:1091–1097	720 Multi-center	Esomeprazole 40 mg twice daily	16 wks	Improved PEF in subjects with GER and nocturnal asthma symptoms
Sharma B et al.[61] *World J Gastroenterol.* 2007;13(11): 1706–1710	198 Single-site + pH	Omeprazole 20 mg twice daily; domperidone 10 mg three times daily	16 wks	Improved daytime and nighttime asthma symptoms, AM and PM PEF, FEV_1 and FVC, and decreased use of rescue medications
dos Santos LH et al.[60] *J Bras Pneumol.* 2007;33:119–127	44 Single-site + pH	Pantoprazole 40 mg daily	12 wks	Improved asthma symptom scores and QOL; no change in PEF

FEV_1 = Forced expiratory volume in 1 second; FVC = Forced vital capacity; GER = Gastroesophageal reflux; PEF = Peak expiratory flow; PFT = Pulmonary function test; QOL = Quality of life.

asthmatics are more likely to improve with aggressive PPI therapy.[58,59]

Two investigations utilized esophageal pH testing for defining GER.[60,61] dos Santos et al[60] evaluated 35 asthmatics with abnormal esophageal acid contact times with pantoprazole 40 mg daily for 12 weeks, noting an improvement in asthma symptoms and quality of life scores. However, no improvement was noted in PEF.[60] In another large study performed at a single site, Sharma et al[61] utilized both omeprazole, 20 mg twice daily, and domperidone 10 mg three times daily in 198 asthmatics with abnormal esophageal acid contact times for 16 weeks. There was improvement in daytime and nighttime asthma symptoms as well as morning and evening PEF. Furthermore, there were improvements in FEV_1 and FVC, and a decrease in the number of asthma rescue dose inhalations required for asthma control. This study used both acid suppression and a prokinetic agent which led the investigators to hypothesize that in carefully selected asthmatics, the addition of a prokinetic agent may also decrease nonacid reflux.[61] They did not utilize esophageal impedance testing in their study.[61]

Uncontrolled surgical trials also examined asthma outcomes. In 110 carefully selected asthmatics with GER undergoing fundoplication, approximately one-third of subjects were free of asthma symptoms, and another 40% had asthma symptom improvement.[3] Both open and laparoscopic fundoplication procedures showed similar results in controlling asthma symptoms. Many trials had design flaws and did not monitor GER and asthma outcomes in a standardized way.[62]

Two placebo-controlled trials compared surgical versus medical GER therapy in asthmatics with GER; however, both trials were performed before the availability of PPIs.[63,64] Larrain and colleagues[63] examined 81 nonallergic asthmatics with GER, with a minimum follow up period of 6 months. Asthma symptoms improved by 74% in the medically-treated group utilizing cimetidine 300 mg four times daily, and by 77% in the surgically treated group.[63] In a 2-year follow-up study, Sontag et al[64] evaluated 62 asthmatics with GER who were randomized to receive either antacid (placebo), ranitidine (150 mg three times daily), or surgical fundoplication. Only the surgically treated group had significant improvement in asthma symptoms, asthma medication use, and pulmonary function tests.[64]

In conclusion, aggressive GER therapy does not improve asthma outcomes in the general asthma population; however, selected patients, especially those with GER symptoms, show improvement. The findings may be more pronounced in asthmatics with abnormal esophageal acid contact times. Furthermore, asthma symptoms are more likely to improve than pulmonary function in response to aggressive medical GER therapy. Potential asthma variables that predict asthma response include the presence of nonallergic asthma, oral corticosteroid use, LABA use, nighttime asthma symptoms, and/or reflux-associated asthma symptoms.[18,58-60,63] Gastroesophageal reflux variables that predict asthma response with GER therapy include the presence of regurgitation and/or abnormal amounts of esophageal acid at the proximal esophageal pH probe.[56] These potential predictors need to be validated in prospective trials.

DIAGNOSTIC AND GER MANAGEMENT STRATEGIES

Since aggressive GER therapy may improve asthma outcomes in selected individuals, asthmatics should be screened for the presence of GER. Currently, there is no diagnostic test available that accurately diagnoses GER-triggered asthma. As GER can potentially cause asthmalike symptoms in patients without asthma, patients should be carefully evaluated for the presence of asthma by performing pulmonary function tests, methacholine challenge tests, and other asthma diagnostic strategies as recommended by the National Heart Lung and Blood Institute's *Guidelines for the Diagnosis and Management of Asthma*.[1] Furthermore, Di Lorenzo et al[65] compared mild asthmatics with subjects with asthmalike symptoms caused by GER and noted that methacholine challenge tests (airway reactivity of PD_{20} <1500 mcg) and eosinophil count >1% in induced sputum differentiated mild asthmatics from subjects with asthmalike symptoms caused by GER.

Although prospective trials are needed to assess the diagnostic accuracy of an empiric 3-month PPI GER treatment trial in asthmatics, it can be used to identify individual asthmatics with GER-triggered asthma.[3] Twice-daily dosing, an hour before breakfast and dinner, is recommended for a period of at least 3 months. During this time, asthma outcomes (including asthma symptoms, asthma medication use, PEF, and pulmonary function tests) should be monitored. If an asthmatic has improvement with GER therapy, then continuation of the PPI should be considered. The PPI could be tapered to a once-daily regimen. Empiric GER treatment trials should be considered in asthmatics with moderate to severe persistent asthma, especially in those requiring oral corticosteroid therapy.[3] An American Thoracic Society workshop suggested that GER should be investigated in asthmatics with refractory asthma.[66] Esophageal pH testing should be considered in the asthma nonresponders to PPI therapy to see if esophageal acid is adequately controlled.[3] If esophageal acid is controlled on esophageal pH testing, then two possibilities should be considered. First, that the asthmatic has GER; however, GER is not a potential trigger of their asthma, nor does it impact their asthma. The other possibility is that nonacid reflux may be present and could be influencing airway responsiveness. This is most likely a rare possibility; however, there is minimal data evaluating this possibility. Esophageal diagnostic testing is also strongly recommended prior to considering surgical GER therapy.[3] Surgical fundoplication could be considered in asthmatics whose asthma improves with medical GER therapy, especially in asthmatics with normal esophageal motility and reduced LES pressure.[3] At this time, surgery is not recommended for an asthma indication in the PPI nonresponders.

UNANSWERED QUESTIONS

There are many controversies and unanswered questions about the association between asthma and GER. Currently, there is no diagnostic test that identifies patients with GER-triggered asthma. Preliminary work is being done utilizing exhaled breath condensate biomarker analysis, including pH, as a potential diagnostic test.[67] Although esophageal acid can initiate asthma symptoms, it is difficult to establish a definite cause and effect relationship between GER and asthma. Pathophysiologic mechanisms help establish this association, but much work needs to be done to further define this association.

Another controversy is whether to utilize an empiric PPI trial in asthmatics who do not have GER symptoms. Kiljander et al[59] noted that asthma symptoms and PEF did not improve in asthmatics who did not have GER symptoms. One hopes carefully designed prospective trials will answer this controversy.

Another unanswered question is whether nonacid GER can trigger asthma.[68] As currently available medical therapy for GER does not definitively control nonacid GER, fundoplication may be necessary.[69] Also, there are minimal data available examining long-term GER management in asthmatics with GER-triggered asthma. One hopes future investigations will offer guidance to these unanswered questions.

CONCLUSIONS

Multiple investigations show a strong association between GER and asthma. Furthermore, aggressive treatment of

GER can improve asthma outcomes in selected asthmatics. Data suggest that GER is more common in asthmatics in population-based studies, incidence studies, and cohort studies of consecutive asthmatics. Furthermore, esophageal acid can elicit airway responses through multiple pathophysiologic mechanisms. Placebo-controlled randomized studies show that asthma symptoms improve with medical GER therapy, although marked improvements in pulmonary function may not occur. Subsets of asthmatics are more likely to improve and further work needs to be done to examine the predictors of asthma response and identify those asthmatics with GER-triggered asthma.

Acknowledgment. I acknowledge the kind editorial assistance of Arren Graf in the preparation of this manuscript.

REFERENCES

1. Expert Panel Report 3 (EPR-3): *Guidelines for the Diagnosis and Management of Asthma—Summary Report 2007*. National Institutes of Health, National Heart, Lung, and Blood Institute, NIH Publication No. 08-5846. October 2007.
2. Sontag SJ, Harding SM. Gastroesophageal reflux and asthma. In: Goyal RK, Shaker R, eds. *Goyal and Shaker's GI Motility Online.* New York, NY: Nature Publishing Group; 2006. doi:10.1038/gimo 47 Retrieved 1-23-08 from: http://www.nature.com/gimo/contents/pt1/full/gimo47.html
3. Harding SM. Gastroesophageal reflux: a potential asthma trigger. *Immunol Allergy Clin North Am.* 2005;25:131-148.
4. Moorman JE, Rudd RA, Johnson CA, et al. Centers for Disease Control and Prevention. National surveillance for asthma—United States, 1980-2004. *MMWR Surveill Summ.* 2007;56(8):1-54.
5. Harding SM. Gastroesophageal reflux and asthma: insight into the association. *J Allergy Clin Immunol.* 1999;104(2 pt 1); 251-259.
6. El-Serag HB, Sonnenberg A. Comorbid occurrence of laryngeal or pulmonary disease with esophagitis in United States military veterans. *Gastroenterology.* 1997; 113(3):755-760.
7. Hancox RJ, Poulton R, Taylor DR, et al. Associations between respiratory symptoms, lung function and gastro-oesophageal reflux symptoms in a population-based birth cohort. *Respir Res.* 2006;7:142-151.
8. Nordenstedt H, Nilsson M, Johansson S, et al. The relation between gastroesophageal reflux and respiratory symptoms in a population-based study. The Nord-Trøndelag Health Survey. *Chest.* 2006; 129(4):1051-1056.
9. Ruigómez A, Rodríguez LA, Wallander MA, Johansson S, Thomas M, Price D. Gastroesophageal reflux disease and asthma: a longitudinal study in UK general practice. *Chest.* 2005;128(1):85-93.
10. Field SK, Underwood M, Brant R, Cowie RL. Prevalence of gastroesophageal reflux symptoms in asthma. *Chest.* 1996; 109(2):316-322.
11. Kiljander TO, Laitinen JO. The prevalence of gastroesophageal reflux disease in adult asthmatics. *Chest.* 2004;126(5): 1490-1494.
12. Kjellén G, Brundin A, Tibbling L, Wranne B. Oesophageal function in asthmatics. *Eur J Respir Dis.* 1981;62(2):87-94.
13. Sontag SJ, O'Connell S, Khandelwal S, et al. Most asthmatics have gastroesophageal reflux with or without bronchodilator therapy. *Gastroenterology.* 1990;99(3): 613-620.
14. Sontag SJ, Schnell TG, Miller TQ, et al. Prevalence of oesophagitis in asthmatics. *Gut.* 1992;33(7):872-876.
15. Harding SM, Guzzo MR, Richter JE. 24-hour esophageal pH testing in asthmatics. Respiratory symptom correlation with

esophageal acid events. *Chest.* 1999; 115(3):654-659.
16. Harding SM. The prevalence of gastroesophageal reflux in asthma patients without reflux symptoms. *Am J Respir Crit Care Med.* 2000;162(3):34-39.
17. ten Brinke A, Sterk PJ, Masclee AA, et al. Risk factors of frequent exacerbations in difficult-to-treat asthma. *Eur Respir J.* 2005;26(5):812-818.
18. Irwin RS, Curley FJ, French CL. Difficult-to-control asthma: contributing factors and outcome of a systematic management protocol. *Chest.* 1993;103(6):1662-1669.
19. Harding SM. GERD, airway disease, and the mechanisms of interaction. In: Stein MR, ed. *Gastroesophageal Reflux Disease and Airway Disease. Lung Biology in Health and Disease.* Vol 129. New York, NY: Marcel Dekker, Inc; 1999:139-178.
20. Lodi U, Harding SM, Coghlan HC, Guzzo MR, Walker LH. Autonomic regulation in asthmatics with gastroesophageal reflux. *Chest.* 1997;111(1):65-70.
21. Mittal RK, Balaban DH. The esophagogastric junction. *N Engl J Med.* 1997; 336(13):924-932.
22. Roussos C, Macklem PT. The respiratory muscles. *N Engl J Med.* 1982;307(13): 786-797.
23. Ekström T, Tibbling L. Influence of theophylline on gastro-oesophageal reflux and asthma. *Eur J Clin Pharmacol.* 1988;35(4):353-356.
24. DiMarino AJ, Cohen S. Effect of an oral beta2-adrenergic agonist on lower esophageal sphincter pressure in normals and in patients with achalasia. *Dig Dis Sci.* 1982;27(12):1063-1066.
25. Crowell MD, Zayat EN, Lacy BE, Schetter-Duncan A, Liu MC. The effects of an inhaled beta(2)-adrenergic agonist on lower esophageal function: a dose response study. *Chest.* 2001;120(4):1184-1189.
26. Lazenby JP, Guzzo MR, Harding SM, Patterson PE, Johnson LF, Bradley LA. Oral corticosteroids increase esophageal acid contact times in patients with stable asthma. *Chest.* 2002;121(4):625-634.
27. Gunnbjörnsdóttir MI, Omenaas E, Gislason T, et al. RHINE Study Group. Obesity and nocturnal gastro-oesophageal reflux are related to onset of asthma and respiratory symptoms. *Eur Respir J.* 2004; 24(1):116-121.
28. Mansfield LE, Stein MR. Gastroesophageal reflux and asthma: a possible reflex mechanism. *Ann Allergy.* 1978;41(4):224-226.
29. Mansfield LE, Hameister HH, Spaulding HS, Smith NJ, Glab N. The role of the vagus nerve in airway narrowing caused by intraesophageal hydrochloric acid provocation and esophageal distention. *Ann Allergy.* 1981;47(6):431-434.
30. Wright RA, Miller SA, Corsello BF. Acid-induced esophagobronchial-cardiac reflexes in humans. *Gastroenterology.* 1990;99(1):71-73.
31. Schan CA, Harding SM, Haile JM, Bradley LA, Richter JE. Gastroesophageal reflux-induced bronchoconstriction. An intraesophageal acid infusion study using state-of-the-art technology. *Chest.* 1994; 106(3):731-737.
32. Harding SM, Schan CA, Guzzo MR, Alexander RW, Bradley LA, Richter JE. Gastroesophageal reflux-induced bronchoconstriction. Is microaspiration a factor? *Chest.* 1995;108(5):1220-1227.
33. Harding SM, Guzzo MR, Maples RV, Alexander RW, Richter JE. Gastroesophageal reflux induced bronchoconstriction: vagolytic doses of atropine diminish airway responses to esophageal acid infusion [Abstract]. *Am J Respir Crit Care Med.* 1995;151:A589.
34. Fischer A, Canning JB, Undem JB, Kummer W. Evidence for an esophageal origin of VIP-IR and NO synthase-IR nerves innervating the guinea pig trachealis: a retrograde neuronal tracing and immunohistochemical analysis. *J Comp Neurol.* 1998;394(3):326-334.
35. Hamamoto J, Kohrogi H, Kawano O, et al. Esophageal stimulation by hydrochloric acid causes neurogenic inflammation in the airways in guinea pigs. *J Appl Physiol.* 1997;82(3):738-745.

36. Vincent D, Cohen-Jonathan AM, Leport J, et al. Gastro-oesophageal reflux prevalence and relationship with bronchial reactivity in asthma. *Eur Respir J.* 1997; 10(10):2255-2259.
37. Hervé P, Denjean A, Jian R, Simmoneau G, Duroux P. Intraesophageal perfusion of acid increases the bronchomotor response to methacholine and to isocapnic hyperventilation in asthmatic subjects. *Am Rev Respir Dis.* 1986;134(5): 986-989.
38. Ferrari M, Benini L, Brotto E, et al. Omeprazole reduces the response to capsaicin but not to methacholine in asthmatic patients with proximal reflux. *Scand J Gastroenterol.* 2007;42(3): 299-307.
39. Cuttitta G, Cibella F, Visconti A, Scichilone N, Belia V, Bonsignore G. Spontaneous gastroesophageal reflux and airway patency during the night in adult asthmatics. *Am J Respir Crit Care Med.* 2000;161(1):177-181.
40. Tuchman DN, Boyle JT, Pack AI, et al. Comparison of airway responses following tracheal or esophageal acidification in the cat. *Gastroenterology.* 1984;87(4): 872-881.
41. Sant'Ambrogio FB, Sant'Ambrogio G, Chung K. Effects of HCL-pepsin laryngeal instillations on upper airway patency-maintaining mechanisms. *J Appl Physiol.* 1998;84(4):1229-1304.
42. Jack CI, Calverley PM, Donnelly RJ, et al. Simultaneous tracheal and oesophageal pH measurements in asthmatic patients with gastro-oesophageal reflux. *Thorax.* 1995;50(2):201-204.
43. Wesseling G, Brummer RJ, Wouters EF, ten Velde CP. Gastric asthma? No change in respiratory impedance during intraesophageal acidification in adult asthmatics. *Chest.* 1999;104(6):1733-1736.
44. Field SK. A critical review of the studies of the effects of simulated or real gastroesophageal reflux on pulmonary function in asthmatic adults. *Chest.* 1999;115(3): 848-856.
45. Field SK, Evans JA, Price LM. The effects of acid perfusion of the esophagus on ventilation and respiratory sensation. *Am J Respir Crit Care Med.* 1998;157 (4 pt1):1058-1062.
46. Ricciardolo FL, Gaston B, Hunt J. Acid stress in the pathology of asthma. *J Allergy Clin Immunol.* 2004;113(4): 610-619.
47. Patterson RN, Johnston BT, Ardill JE, Heaney LG, McGarvey LP. Increased tachykinin levels in induced sputum from asthmatic and cough patients with acid reflux. *Thorax.* 2007;62(6):491-495.
48. Silvestri M, Mattioli G, Defillippi AC, et al. Correlations between exhaled nitric oxide and pH-metry data in asthmatics with gastro-oesophageal reflux. *Respiration.* 2004;71(4):329-335.
49. Carpagnano GE, Resta O, Ventura MT, et al. Airway inflammation in subjects with gastro-oesophageal reflux and gastro-oesophageal reflux-related asthma. *J Intern Med.* 2006;259(3):323-331.
50. Shimizu Y, Dobashi K, Zhao JJ, et al. Proton pump inhibitor improves breath markers in moderate asthma with gastro-esophageal reflux disease. *Respiration.* 2007;74(5):558-564.
51. Stein MR. Advances in the approach to gastroesophageal reflux (GER) and asthma. *J Asthma.* 1999;36(4):309-314.
52. Perng DW, Chang KT, Su KC, et al. Exposure of airway epithelium to bile acids associated with gastroesophageal reflux symptoms: a relation to transforming growth factor-beta 1 production and fibroblast proliferation. *Chest.* 2007;132(5): 1548-1556.
53. Field SK, Sutherland LR. Does medical antireflux therapy improve asthma in asthmatics with gastroesophageal reflux?: a critical review of the literature. *Chest.* 1998;114(1):275-283.
54. Coughlan JL, Gibson PG, Henry RL. Medical treatment for reflux oesophagitis does not consistently improve asthma control: a systematic review. *Thorax.* 2001;56(3):198-204.

55. Gibson PG, Henry RL, Coughlan JL. Gastro-oesophageal reflux treatment for asthma in adults and children. *Cochrane Database Syst Rev.* 2003;(2):CD001496.
56. Harding SM, Richter JE, Guzzo MR, Schan CA, Alexander RW, Bradley LA. Asthma and gastroesophageal reflux: acid suppressive therapy improves asthma outcome. *Am J Med.* 1996;100(4):395–405.
57. Boeree MJ, Peters FT, Postma DS, Kleibeuker JH. No effects of high-dose omeprazole in patients with severe airway hyperresponsiveness and (a)symptomatic gastro-oesophageal reflux. *Eur Respir J.* 1998;11(5):1070–1074.
58. Littner MR, Leung FW, Ballard ED 2nd, Huang B, Samra NK. Lansoprazole Asthma Study Group. Effects of 24 weeks of lansoprazole therapy on asthma symptoms, exacerbations, quality of life, and pulmonary function in adult asthmatic patients with acid reflux symptoms. *Chest.* 2005; 128(3):1128–1135.
59. Kiljander TO, Harding SM, Field SK, et al. Effects of esomeprazole 40 mg twice daily on asthma: a randomized placebo-controlled trial. *Am J Respir Crit Care Med.* 2006;173(10):1091–1097.
60. dos Santos LH, Ribeiro IO, Sanchez PG, Hetzel JL, Felicetti JC, Cardoso PF. Evaluation of pantoprazole treatment response of patients with asthma and gastro-esophageal reflux: a randomized prospective double-blind placebo-controlled study. *J Bras Pneumol.* 2007;33(2): 119–127.
61. Sharma B, Sharma M, Daga MK, Sachdev GK, Bondi E. Effect of omeprazole and domperidone on adult asthmatics with gastroesophageal reflux. *World J Gastroenterol.* 2007;13(11):1706–1710.
62. Field SK, Gelfand GA, McFadden SD. The effects of antireflux surgery on asthmatics with gastroesophageal reflux. *Chest.* 1999;116(3):766–774.
63. Larrain A, Carrasco E, Galleguillos F, Sepulveda R, Pope CE 2nd. Medical and surgical treatment of nonallergic asthma associated with gastroesophageal reflux. *Chest.* 1991;99(6):1330–1335.
64. Sontag SJ, O'Connell S, Khandelwal S, et al. Asthmatics with gastroesophageal reflux: long term results of a randomized trial of medical and surgical antireflux therapies. *Am J Gastroenterol.* 2003; 98(5):987–999.
65. Di Lorenzo G, Mansueto P, Esposito-Pellitteri M, et al. The characteristics of different diagnostic tests in adult mild asthmatic patients: comparison with patients with asthma-like symptoms by gastro-oesophageal reflux. *Respir Med.* 2007;101(7):1455–1461.
66. Proceedings of the ATS workshop on refractory asthma: current understand, recommendations, and unanswered questions. American Thoracic Society. *Am J Respir Crit Care Med.* 2000;162(6): 2341–2351.
67. Hunt J. Exhaled breath condensate pH assays. *Immunol Allergy Clin North Am.* 2007;27(4):597–606.
68. Shay S, Tutuian R, Sifrim D, et al. Twenty-four hour ambulatory simultaneous impedance and pH monitoring: a multicenter report of normal values from 60 healthy volunteers. *Am J Gastroenterol.* 2004; 99(6):1037–1043.
69. Irwin RS, Zawacki JK, Wilson MM, French CT, Callery MP. Chronic cough due to gastroesophageal reflux disease: failure to resolve despite total/near-total elimination of esophageal acid. *Chest.* 2002; 121(4):1132–1140.

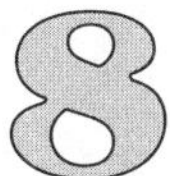

Gastroesophageal Reflux Disease and Cough: An Evidence-Based Approach to Diagnosis and Treatment

J. Matthew Bohning and Joel E. Richter

Gastroesophageal reflux disease (GERD) is widely recognized as one of the most common diseases in the western world. Typical signs and symptoms (ie, heartburn, regurgitation, erosive esophagitis) are well described, readily diagnosed, and are very responsive to acid suppression therapy. A variety of extraesophageal symptoms are attributed to GERD including most commonly cough, laryngopharyngitis, hoarseness, and asthma, as well as subglottic stenosis, pulmonary fibrosis, globus, otitis, sinusitis, and sleep apnea. In the absence of typical reflux symptoms, these symptoms are more problematic in their relationship to GERD and, therefore, to treat effectively. Although some patient complaints definitely are due to acid reflux, there are many other causes for these nondigestive symptoms including smoking, alcohol, voice abuse, postnasal drip, allergies, sinusitis, and reactive airway disease. This diagnostic quandary has led to much debate about the role of GERD in these symptoms, and the most effective means of diagnosis and treatment.

Although there is a high prevalence of extraesophageal symptoms in patients with GERD, it is unclear whether these symptoms are entirely caused by acid reflux. In the ProGERD study by Jaspersen et al[1] (a prospective multicenter open cohort study following 6,215 patients with GERD treated with esopmeprazole), 31% of patients with nonerosive disease, and 35% of patients with erosive disease had at least one extraesophageal complaint. A population-based study from Olmsted County, Minnesota, using a validated questionnaire, reported that 59% of the population had typical reflux symptoms sometime over the course of a year.[2] Although 80% of patients with frequent GERD reported atypical symptoms (including non-cardiac chest pain and dysphagia, but not cough), 49% reported atypical symptoms with no heartburn or regurgitation. This high prevalence of extraesophageal symptoms in patients without typical reflux complaints illustrates the broad overlap that symptom complexes may have and emphasizes the diagnostic dilemma: Is GERD to blame for these atypical symptoms without typical reflux symptoms (silent GERD), or is there another process separate from acid reflux that is responsible?

This narrative review offers a critical evaluation of the literature, and provides an algorithm for the diagnosis and treatment of cough and GERD based on the available data.

EPIDEMIOLOGY

Cough is one of the most common presenting symptoms to family practitioners,[3] responsible for 26 million office visits to physicians each year,[4] and is frequently a reason for referral to pulmonologists and otolaryngologists. The prevalence of GERD as a cause of cough extrapolated from treatment studies varies from 5% to 41%. Irwin reports an increasing prevalence, from 21% in 1990[5] (third most common cause) to 36% in 1998,[6] second only to postnasal drip.

The first report from Irwin et al in 1990[5] prospectively evaluated 102 patients with cough using a previously validated diagnostic protocol, including esophageal pH monitoring. The cause of cough was identified in 99% of patients, leading to a remarkable 98% successful treatment rate with therapy tailored to the identified cause. GERD was identified as causing the cough in 28% of patients by symptoms, barium swallow, or esophageal pH monitoring. Cough was the only manifestation of GERD in 41% of these patients, implying that many patients had "silent" reflux. In this study 73% of patients had only one identifiable cause of cough. Unfortunately, the diagnosis of GERD was not standardized nor consistent; among the 28 patients in the GERD group, two did not have any objective study diagnosing GERD, eight did not have pH monitoring, and only five had both positive barium study and esophageal monitoring. The lack of standardization, variability in positive studies, and probably high placebo treatment response makes these data difficult to interpret.

The later study by French and Irwin[6] was designed to assess the impact of chronic cough on quality of life, not the etiology of cough. Only 28 patients were enrolled in this study. Using the same diagnostic protocol as in their earlier study, the authors found that 36% of patients had GERD as the cause of cough. All patients responded to aggressive medical therapy consisting of "high protein, low fat antireflux diet, eating three meals a day, not eating or drinking 2 to 3 hours prior to lying down except for taking medications, head of bed elevation, and metoclopramide and/or H2-blockers." It is unclear why PPIs were not more commonly used in their 1992 study, nor do the authors specify exactly what medication dose/frequency/combination was used. In stark contrast to their earlier study, 93% of patients were found to have *more* than one cause of their cough. Here, again, there may have been a significant placebo response not elicited in this noncontrolled study.

In another small, but placebo-controlled study designed to evaluate the role of esophageal pH testing and omeprazole in the diagnosis of chronic cough, Ours et al[7] observed a GERD prevalence of only 8%. Seventy-one patients with unexplained cough were evaluated, with other causes being identified in 48 patients. The remaining 23 patients had esophageal pH monitoring and, independent to their test results, were randomized to omeprazole BID versus placebo. Patients with negative pH testing did not respond to PPI therapy, whereas only 6/17 (26%) patients with abnormal pH studies had marked improvement in their cough after 3 months of omeprazole therapy.

Based on this limited and conflicting data, the prevalence of GER as a *primary* cause of cough is still poorly defined. We believe it is probably responsible for no more than 10 to 20% of patients, at best. Larger, randomized, controlled treatment studies are needed to adequately assess the true prevalence of GERD in cough.

PATHOPHYSIOLOGY

The role of acid reflux in initiating and perpetuating a cough is multifactorial (Fig 8-1). Coughing is a complicated coordination of stimulation, sensory input and integration, and respiratory muscle motor activity. Animal studies have found that the cough reflex is initiated by vagal afferent nerves.[8] Acid reflux is hypothesized to induce cough either by direct irritation or microaspiration stimulating

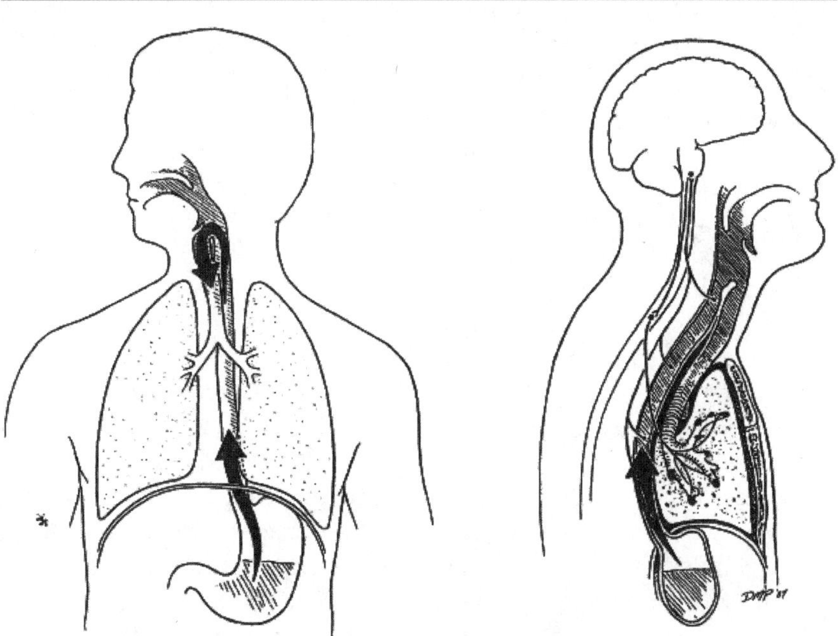

Fig 8–1. Potential pathophysiologic mechanism by which GERD may cause cough. *Left:* Aspiration of gastric refluxate irritating the larynx and lungs. *Right:* An esophageal-bronchial reflux via the vagus nerve. *Am J Gastroenterol.* 2000;95(suppl):S11.

the airway afferent nerves, or possibly by affecting the esophageal vagal afferent nerves. Studies have demonstrated that mucus secretion, bronchospasm, and cough can be stimulated by the stomach or esophageal afferent nerves.[9] The presence of acid in the esophagus may also sensitize the cough reflex. Ing et al[10] showed that patients with pH-proven GERD and cough were more sensitive to intraesophageal HCl infusion than healthy controls, with more frequent coughing and cough episodes. Another small physiology study by Wu et al[11] demonstrated that infusion of HCl into the distal esophagus significantly increased cough responsiveness to capsaisin in patients with mild persistent asthma.[12] These effects are probably due to synergistic interactions between esophageal nociceptors and airway sensory nerves which both terminate in the same regions of the nucleus of the solitary tract in the central nervous system[9]; this effect can be reduced by vagotomy.[8]

The amount of acid needed to induce cough is uncertain. Unlike the esophagus, the pharynx lacks an acid clearance mechanism, and is more vulnerable to injury. Thus, a small amount of acid may cause irritation and evoke symptoms. Even physiologic amounts of acid exposure may be enough to cause cough in susceptible patients, but treatment trials with acid suppression medications have mixed results. Acid reflux may also be an innocent bystander in chronic cough, with reflux *resulting* from coughing due to increased intra-abdominal pressure forcing gastric contents retrograde across the LES. This can contribute to a vicious cycle of cough and reflux and adds to the dilemma of which came first: acid reflux or cough?

DIAGNOSTIC TESTING

Guidelines have been proposed by several societies to aid in the diagnosis of cough and GERD, but none are universally accepted. The high frequency of both GERD and cough among the population makes a definitive diagnosis difficult. Although acid reflux disease may be diagnosed relatively easily, its causal relationship with cough may not be as readily deduced. Compulsive history taking is an important first step in the evaluation of patients with chronic cough. Many causes of chronic cough other than GERD can be identified by history alone, including postnasal drip, smoking, asthma, and medications (such as ACEi inhibitors). If possible causes are identified, a trial of decongestants, antihistamines, bronchodilators, smoking cessation, or medication withdrawal can be both diagnostic and therapeutic. A combination of tests including laryngoscopy, endoscopy, pH monitoring, barium studies, manometry, and impedance testing, as well as medical therapy trials with proton-pump inhibitors (PPIs), often are required to identify whether or not GERD is causing the cough.

Laryngoscopy and Endoscopy

Laryngoscopy and endoscopy provide direct evidence of irritation to the larynx and esophagus. Although erosive esophagitis seen on endoscopy correlates well with GERD, the finding of "reflux laryngitis" and its extrapolation to implicating proximal reflux as a cause of cough is much less specific. A large randomized placebo controlled study by Vaezi et al[12] looking at the treatment of chronic posterior laryngitis with esomeprazole illustrates this point well. Patients in the study underwent screening laryngoscopy and the laryngeal findings were graded by experienced otolaryngologists using an agreed on chronic posterior laryngitis index. This visual grading system included the findings of posterior surface erythema and edema, arytenoid mucosa erythema, surface irregularities, and vocal fold erythema and edema. Despite all patients having abnormal laryngeal exams, only 29% (19/65 patients) had pH-documented reflux using a triple-pH probe. Furthermore, these patients with suspected "reflux laryngitis" did no better on esomeprazole 40 mg BID for 12 weeks than on placebo, confirming the lack of specificity of these findings and GERD-related disease.

Poelmans et al[13] examined the yield of EGD in 405 PPI naïve patients in Belgium with suspected reflux related chronic ear, nose, and throat symptoms, including 117 with nonproductive cough. Only 20% had classic reflux symptoms, but surprisingly 52% of patients had erosive esophagitis on EGD. All patients subsequently received H2 blockers or PPI therapy. Patients with erosive esophagitis responded significantly better than those without esophagitis at 2, 4, and 8 weeks of treatment, but not by the end of the 16-week study. Among all patients, the subgroup with nonproductive cough had the best benefit, with "good symptomatic" response in nearly 90% of patients. Based on this study, the authors suggested that endoscopic evidence of esophagitis confirms an acid reflux cause for chronic cough resulting in a good response to PPI therapy. However, the treatment regimen was not placebo controlled, and this PPI naïve patient population is not typical of patients seen in specialty clinics in the United States.

ESOPHAGEAL PH MONITORING

The gold standard for diagnosing GERD is catheter-based 24-hour pH monitoring. A pH sensor located 5 cm above the manometrically identified lower esophageal sphincter detects the acidity of the surrounding fluid. Normally occurring acid exposure is defined as a pH of <4 for no more than 4.5% to 5.5% of the total 24-hour period. More recently, the BRAVO (Medtronic, Minneapolis, Minn.) wireless capsule was developed. After being attached to the esophageal mucosa 6 cm proximal to the squamocolumnar junction, the pH probe transmits a signal to a remote pack worn by the patient. This more "friendly" pH-probe avoids the transnasal catheter, is unobtrusive and has the ability to record data for 48 hours or more while the patient performs normal daily activities, potentially giving greater insight into reflux patterns and their relationship to daily activities.[14]

Some studies employ dual-probe pH catheters to determine the relationship between distal and proximal reflux and atypical GERD symptoms. In a dual-pH system, the distal probe is placed in the customary 5 cm location above the LES, while the proximal pH probe is usually placed just above the upper esophageal sphincter. In theory, patients with extra-esophageal symptoms (cough, asthma, laryngopharyngitis) should have simultaneous evidence of both distal and more proximal reflux, especially if microaspiration is causing the symptoms. Unfortunately, most studies find a poor correlation between proximal reflux and symptoms. In a study of 12 patients referred for cough likely due to GERD after a standard diagnostic workup, the authors concluded that distal acid reflux occurred more frequently, and induced significantly more coughs than did proximal reflux.[15] However, there was extreme variability of both reflux and coughing episodes among patients; some patients had no coughs due to reflux whereas others had 100% of coughs due to reflux. This heterogeneity resulted in extremely large standard deviations around the averaged data and may confound the results. In the Vaezi et al[12] study, all patients had some type of extraesophageal complaint (throat clearing, cough, hoarseness, globus, sore throat), but there was no evidence that pharyngeal acid reflux had any association with the nature of the primary symptom or symptom severity.

This illustrates some of the problems with traditional pH testing. As described previously, even small amounts of esophageal acid exposure, including "normal" distal acid exposure, may provoke cough. Thus, the interpretation of a "negative" study is less clear. Given the single-pH sensor in conventional pH monitoring, traditional pH testing also cannot distinguish antegrade from retrograde acidity, possibly confounding the interpretation of pH findings. pH testing would also not be helpful in diagnosing nonacid reflux events, such as bile reflux. Finally, the lack of a sophisticated cough monitor precludes defining with consistency the relationship between cough and GERD.

Impedance/pH Monitoring

Impedance has been used in conjunction with manometry and pH monitoring in the diagnosis of GERD. Impedance changes with the resistance of the material in contact with the sensors. Liquids such as water and acid have a low impedance relative to the esophageal mucosa, while air has a high impedance. Combined with manometry and pH monitoring, this may be helpful in distinguishing antegrade (swallowed acidic beverages or food) from retrograde reflux, uncovering motility disturbances, and in identifying nonacid reflux. Zerbib et al[16] correlated simultaneous pH-impedance monitoring in 150 patients (79 off PPI therapy, 71 on therapy) with a variety of symptoms possibly related to GERD, including 62 with cough. A positive symptom association probability (SAP) was defined as a symptom occurring within 5 minutes of a liquid reflux event measured by impedance. Overall, 47% (63/134) of symptomatic patients had a positive SAP, 41 patients in the group off PPI therapy, and 22 in the group on PPI therapy. Of these 63 patients, 13 had nonacid reflux associated with symptoms, but only 3/41 (7%) in the group off therapy. This implies that the addition of impedance adds little diagnostic value compared to pH monitoring alone in patients not taking a PPI. The diagnostic yield was greater, however, in the group taking PPIs, finding that 10/22 (46%) patients had symptoms possibly due to nonacid reflux.

Sifrim et al[17] specifically examined the association of cough and reflux with simultaneous pH-manometry-impedance monitoring in 22 patients referred for cough of unknown etiology. Cough was objectively defined manometrically as phasic, short, rapid pressure rises occurring simultaneously and with the same pressure configuration at all manometric recording sites. This technique allows accurate assessment of the cough event to pH drops. Most cough episodes (70%) were not related to reflux events. Among the 198 cough episodes (30%) occurring within a 2-minute window around a reflux episode, 49% of cough episodes were preceded by reflux, whereas 51% of coughs were *followed* by reflux. Among the 98 reflux-cough episodes, 65% involved acid reflux (pH <4), 29% involved weakly acidic reflux (4<pH<7), and 6% involved weakly alkaline reflux (pH >7). Unfortunately, this study was only a physiologic evaluation, with an unknown outcome of cough with acid suppression therapy.

Tutuian et al[18] specifically examined multi-channel intraluminal impedance (MII)-pH monitoring in 50 patients with persistent cough despite twice-daily PPIs, with or without nocturnal H2RAs. A symptom index (SI) was considered positive if at least half of the cough episodes, as recorded by a diary, were preceded by reflux within a 5-minute window. Only 26% of patients had a positive SI; however, all patients with a positive SI had nonacid reflux. Of these 13 patients, 6 underwent laparoscopic Nissen fundoplication. Of the five patients available for phone survey at a median follow-up of 17 months, all were asymptomatic and not receiving PPI therapy. The higher incidence of non-acid reflux in this group compared to the Sifrim study is likely due to the use of PPIs and the inherent inclusion bias. Unfortunately, cough episodes were recorded by patient diary, and the authors did not comment on the number of cough→reflux episodes. This study does reinforce one point: Given maximal medical acid suppression, persistent cough is likely due to some other reason than acidic gastroesophageal reflux, possibly nonacid reflux.

Thus, impedance combined with pH and manometric monitoring may be beneficial in diagnosing cough due to reflux, particularly nonacid reflux in patients taking PPIs, but results should be temporally related to symptoms. Furthermore, pH studies not utilizing an accurate "cough monitor" may overestimate the episodes of coughing preceded by reflux episodes.

Other Diagnostic Tests

Several other modalities are used to diagnose GERD and help determine the etiology of chronic cough. The diagnosis of GERD is made on barium studies by fluoroscopically observing barium spontaneously reflux into the esophagus, identifying a hiatal hernia, or inducing reflux with the water siphon test. This is an acceptable diagnostic criteria for GERD in some reported studies but may not be accurate. Johnston et al[19] compared barium findings with esophageal pH monitoring in 125 patients. They found the sensitivity of spontaneous reflux and hiatus hernia were low (26% and 43%, respectively), and specificities only modest (77% and 65%, respectively). Although the addition of a water-siphon test increased the sensitivity to 92%, the specificity was zero. Therefore, barium studies should not be solely relied on to diagnose GERD.

Bronchoscopy can help determine the etiology of chronic cough by direct observation of the larynx and upper airway and by performing biopsy, lavage, and aspiration. Barnes et al[21] evaluated the utility of flexible bronchoscopy in the evaluation of 48 patients with chronic cough. Bronchoscopy aided little in the diagnosis of cough, and did not result in successful treatment alterations. Of these 48 patients, one patient had minimal arytenoids redundancy and responded to GERD treatment.

TREATMENT STUDIES

A comprehensive search of the medical literature using PubMed, Google Scholar, and the Cochrane Review database were performed using the following key words: gastroesophageal reflux disease, cough, atypical symptoms, diagnosis, and treatment study. Medical treatment studies were included if the primary therapeutic option was PPIs, and excluded if the study included cisapride (which is not FDA approved in the United States), if a large proportion of patients were primarily treated with H2RAs (which suppress acid much less effectively), or if a separate analysis of cough outcome (in patients with a variety of extraesophageal complaints) was not reported. All surgical studies found from 2000 to 2006 were included if cough was defined as a primary or secondary outcome. In total, 19 studies were found and reviewed in detail: eight studies investigating medical treatment,[7,12,21-26] 10 surgical treatment studies,[27-36] and one Cochrane review[37] (Table 8-1). A total of 1,799 patients were studied (567 and 1,232 in medical and surgical groups, respectively), in a variety of study designs. There were five randomized double-blinded placebo-controlled studies,[7,12,23,25,26] one prospective concurrent controlled study,[35] one randomized nonplacebo-controlled prospective cohort study,[22] eight prospective uncontrolled cohort studies,[24,27,29-33,36] and three uncontrolled retrospective cohort studies.[21,28,34]

Medical Treatment Studies

Medical treatment studies using PPIs have varying results. Four studies of variable designs demonstrate significant improvement in cough with acid suppression therapy[21-24] whereas four others show no difference between medical management with PPIs and placebo.[7,12,25,26]

Positive Studies

Baldi et al[22] found in a nonplacebo controlled randomized prospective cohort (36 patients) study that 60% of patients with cough had complete symptom resolution after both low dose and high dose lansoprazole (30 mg daily plus placebo vs 30 mg BID). All patients were referred by otolaryngologists and pulmonologists after excluding ENT and respiratory causes of chronic cough (methacholine challenge, laryngoscopy, chest x-ray). Patients with possible medication-related cough, smokers, and chronic alcohol users were also excluded. All patients underwent evaluation with symptom assessment, EGD, dual-probe pH monitoring, and were subjected to a prestudy PPI trial for 4 weeks of open label lansoprazole 30 mg. Patients were randomized to daily or twice-daily lansoprazole for 12 weeks if either the EGD or pH data were abnormal, or their cough improved with the PPI test. At the end of the study, 21 of 35 (60%) patients had complete resolution of their cough.

Table 8–1. Select Treatment Study Summary 1999 to 2007 (in order of study design)

Author	Date	Study Type	Treatment	Size	Findings	Comments
Vaezi, M[12]	2006	Prospective randomized, double-blinded, placebo-controlled parallel group	Medical	145	No difference between BID esomeprazole and placebo in symptom, laryngeal signs; poor correlation with laryngoscopy; suggest PPI best determinant of GERD as cause	Atypical patients, all had laryngoscopy, two-catheter three-probe pH (above UES), questionnaire, esomeprazole 40 mg BID vs placebo, 16 week treatment period, follow-up questionnaire and laryngoscopy, pH results skewed by excluded data, but no different between groups (low overall with significant reflux, mod-severe heartburn excluded)
Kiljander, TO[23]	2000	Prospective randomized double-blinded placebo-controlled crossover study	Medical	21	Improved cough and gastric symptom score, but not night-time cough score; group with omeprazole first did not statistically improve until end of placebo period	All with abnormal dual probe pH, only 28% without typical symptoms, did not use cross over data, omeprozole 40 mg daily, questionnaire, 12 week follow-up
Noordzij, JP[25]	2001	Prospective randomized double blinded placebo-controlled study	Medical	30	No significant improvement in subgroup score of cough with PPI or placebo, no improvement in laryngoscopic findings in either group	All patients with abnormal proximal acid exposure (dual probe pH), variety of symptoms including cough (How many?), end of treatment data by questionnaire and laryngoscopy, no follow-up pH data, mixed extraesophageal symptoms
Havas, T[26]	1999	Prospective double-blinded, randomized placebo-controlled	Medical	15	Both placebo and lansoprazole group with improvement in cervical symptoms (including cough) and larygoscopy grading, no statistical difference between the two groups	All patients with abnormal laryngoscopy as entry criteria, had dual-probe pH monitoring/esophageal manometry, EGD, questionnaire; 6 and 12-week follow-up with laryngoscopy and questionnaire; patients with severe erosive esophagitis excluded; only about half had GERD by pH monitoring

continues

Table 8–1. *continued*

Author	Date	Study Type	Treatment	Size	Findings	Comments
Ours, TM[7]	1999	Prospective double-blinded placebo-controlled	Medical	23	35% response to PPI (6/17 with abnormal pH test), No improvement in 6 patients with initially normal pH (though received open label PPI); 26% overall of patients with GERD as etiology of cough; most responded in open-label period after placebo	Excluded other causes; all with dual-probe pH, questionnaire; patients with abnormal pH randomized to placebo vs omeprazole 40 mg BID, then unblinded and open label at 12 weeks, normal pH patients received open-label PPI; post-treatment questionnaire.
Chang, AB[37]	2006	Meta-analysis and systematic review	Medical	11 stds.	Meta-analysis showed no significant difference in primary outcome but trended toward PPI except cough scores in two crossover studies (excludes Vaezi)	Cochrane review (randomized controlled trials with cough as primary outcome and not primarily related to underlying disorder)—Classified based on treatment regimen
Swoger, J[35]	2006	Prospective concurrent controlled study	Surgical	25	1/10 surgical and 1/15 control with symptom improvement, more improvement with treating other causes (asthma/allergy)	All had manometry, dual-probe pH (upper probe 1 cm below UES)/Bilitec on PPI, laryngoscopy; all with abnormal acid exposure off PPI, but normalized on PPI BID; postfundoplication follow-up with BRAVO and laryngoscopy, questionnaire
Baldi, F[22]	2006	Uncontrolled, randomized prospective cohort	Medical	36	60% with complete resolution, no different response rate between the two groups, people with partial response to PPI trial almost 4× as likely to respond (80%/23.1%), no concordance with pH and PPI test	All with endoscopy, pH, PPI test (one positive to be included); questionnaire, randomized to lansoprazole 30 daily with placebo or BID

Author	Date	Study Type	Treatment	Size	Findings	Comments
Dore, MP[24]	2007	Uncontrolled, randomized prospective cohort	Medical	266	69% overall symptom improvement with maximal benefit, number of patients with cough reduced from 65 to 10	Included patients with symptoms or erosive esophagitis; 100 patients in "NERD" group; no objective measurement of pH; symptoms assessed using questionnaire, randomized to one of several BID PPI regimens (rabeprazole, pantoprazole, esomeprazole, lansoprazole) for 3 months
Ekstrom, T[27]	2000	Prospective cohort	Surgical	24	Cough resolved in 45%, day cough improved in 47%, night cough in 80%; asthma improved but not statistically significant	All with cough or asthma, all with hiatal hernia, esophagitis, and abnormal pH (off meds), not responsive to medical therapy (unknown dose)
Farrell, TM[32]	2001	Prospective cohort	Surgical	324	Cough improved in ~97% (resolved ~65%, improved in ~30%), but only 56/324 with cough at baseline. Significant improvement in heartburn in Group 1 compared to Group 2 (99% vs 95%)	Unknown pre-op medical regimen, all with GERD by pH or esophagitis, no objective follow-up, 53-week follow-up with questionnaire, three groups (Group 1 severe typical, minimal atypical, Group 2 severe typical/atypical, Group 3 severe atypical, minimal typical) with all >90% improvement in all symptoms
Novitsky, YW[36]	2002	Prospective cohort	Surgical	21	62% with complete resolution, 14.3% with significant improvement	Patients with "silent GERD," excluded other reasons for cough and aggressive medical therapy (though not BID PPI);

continues

Table 8–1. *continued*

Author	Date	Study Type	Treatment	Size	Findings	Comments
Novitsky, YW[36] *continued*						All had sinus/chest x-ray, barium esophogram, methacholine challenge, bronchoscopy, GES, EGD, dual-probe pH on meds: report 36% cough episodes secondary to distal reflux (acid or alkaline) follow-up questionnaire, 1-year follow-up, no explanation for remaining 64% cough episodes, cough episodes recorded in diary, no objective follow-up data
Wright, RC[30]	2003	Prospective cohort	Surgical	145	92% improvement in postoperative cough	All with hiatal hernia/typical GERD, all patients had Hill repair. Not standardized preoperative screening, unknown pre-op PPI, follow-up with questionnaire alone
Brouwer, R[29]	2003	Prospective cohort	Surgical	29	10/19 pts. with cough had complete resolution, 6 marked, 2 some, 1 no change; 5/11 with wheeze had complete resolution, 5 some, 1 no change; 75% had complete resolution of typical GERD sxs	Good prospective series, all patients with typical symptoms, all on PPI (?dose/frequency), not all with pH/manometry (but then had endoscopic signs of reflux), 650-day follow-up
Rakita, S[33]	2006	Prospective cohort	Surgical	322	69% of cough group (total of 132 patients) with good or excellent outcome; subgroup with severe extraesophageal symptoms but minimal classical symptoms with 70% response	Pre/post operative questionnaire, unknown length of follow-up, no objective postoperative measurement

Author	Date	Study Type	Treatment	Size	Findings	Comments
Duffy, JP[31]	2003	Prospective cohort	Surgical	148	Significant improvement in cough (58%), though lowest response among atypical symptoms	Specifically designed questionnaire (validated?), all with GERD diagnosed by EGD/pH/manometry, barium, unknown pre-operative medical treatment, nearly all with typical symptoms, no objective follow-up data
Vaezi, M[21]	1997	Retrospective cohort	Medical	31	11/31 responded to PPI (10 with abnormal pH), 11/31 responded to pulmonary treatment (2 had abnormal pH but did not respond to PPI), 9 unknown (1 with abnormal pH)	Three groups of chronic cough (GER related, pulmonary related, unknown) defined by response to specific treatment; faster response with PPI, on average 2 months, also with H2 blockers
Thoman, D[28]	2002	Retrospective cohort	Surgical	129	Resolution typical symptoms by 94%, cough by 66% (reduced in 27%)	37 patients with cough, 92 without, significant acid exposure by preoperative pH or endoscopy; patients with other reasons for cough (smoking, ACEi, asthma), unknown response to medical therapy
Greaseon, KL[34]	2002	Retrospective cohort	Surgical	65	Improvement in respiratory symptoms (wheezing 43, sputum 37, cough 30, choking 24, hoarseness 17) (83%), respiratory medications (78%), regurgitation (89%) reflux medications (88%)	Poor retrospective study: not compared to medical treatment, only 16 with pH study, not all with endoscopy, multiple procedure types, not all medically treated before surgery

There was no difference in the response rates between the lansoprazole daily and BID groups. Patients with a partial response to PPIs prior to the trial were nearly four times more likely to respond than those who had no response (80% vs 29%). This remarkable response rate of 60% should not be surprising, considering that 66% (23/35) of patients had a positive PPI trial as an inclusion criteria for this study, effectively enriching their patient population with GERD related cough. Interestingly, there was no correlation between pH monitoring results and PPI response.

A randomized double-blinded placebo-controlled crossover study (21 patients) by Kiljander et al[23] showed significant improvement with omeprazole 40 mg daily for eight weeks in cough and gastric symptom scores, but not nighttime cough scores when compared to placebo. All patients had abnormal pH tests as an inclusion criteria, and only 28% were without typical reflux symptoms. Unfortunately, there was a statistically significant carryover effect after the washout period resulting in the authors excluding the original design in the final analysis. This confounded the data, with each arm acting as conflicting separate trials. The omeprazole-placebo group had significant improvement in cough *only* at the end of the placebo period, whereas the placebo-omeprazole group had significant difference from baseline and end of placebo period compared to end of treatment suggesting a level of spontaneous improvement. Though overall there was significant improvement with daily PPI in this study, the data are not consistent between the two arms.

In a retrospective cohort study examining pH tracings from 31 patients referred for suspected GERD-related cough, Vaezi et al[21] reported a prevalence of 36% and a 100% response rate to varying doses of omeprazole (10 patients) and ranitidine (one patient). These results, however, are misleading. The diagnosis of GERD-related cough was based solely on response to therapy reported by questionnaires. Eleven of the 31 patients (36%) met this criteria, but only 10 had abnormal pH tests. Three other patients had abnormal 24-hour pH testing but did not respond to PPI therapy. It is unclear whether these patients with abnormal pH tests had adequate acid suppression on PPI, possibly leading to a false negative treatment test. The authors concluded that the sensitivity and specificity of 24-hour pH testing was 92% and 82%, respectively, but these numbers should be interpreted with caution given the limitations of the study.

Dore et al[24] studied the effects of various randomly assigned BID PPIs on atypical symptoms as measured by a questionnaire. The study group consisted of 266 patients with heartburn and/or regurgitation, dysphagia, and/or odynophagia, with or without esophagitis. Of these, only 38% had esophagitis but the remainder were thought to have typical reflux symptoms (ie, NERD). No pH monitoring was performed in any of these patients. Overall, 68.4% of patients had "maximum benefit" on treatment, whereas 11.8% had "mild benefit" and 19.8% had "minimum or no benefit." The overall prevalence of cough was significantly reduced after therapy: 65 patients (24.4%) compared to 10 (4.2%). The lack of pH monitoring (especially in this population with a high prevalence of "NERD" patients) and placebo control makes the results of this study difficult to interpret.

A common theme among the studies demonstrating a good response to medical acid suppression therapy was that these cough patients had typical reflux symptoms with abnormal pH tests. Though these studies have flaws, they give credence to the hypothesis that if there is concurrent evidence of classical GERD (typical symptoms, erosive esophagitis, abnormal esophageal pH, and empiric response to PPI) and otherwise unexplained cough, medical acid suppression therapy is more likely to be effective.

Negative Studies

Vaezi et al[12] compared esomeprazole 40 mg BID and placebo in a randomized, double-blinded placebo-controlled study of 145 patients, primarily studying the resolution of symptoms associated with chronic posterior laryngitis defined by a panel of ENT experts. A subgroup of 19 patients had cough as a primary symptom (11 in the treatment group, 8 in the placebo group). All patients were evaluated with symptom questionnaire, standardized laryngoscopy exam, and dual-probe pH monitoring. Patients with moderate to severe heartburn were excluded. There was no statistical difference between the treatment and placebo groups with respect to primary symptom (cough, throat clearing, hoarseness, globus, sore throat) and laryngeal signs seen by laryngoscopy. Among the cough subgroup, patients receiving placebo had a better response than those receiving esomeprazole (25% vs 9%, respectively) although the difference was not statistically significant. A subgroup analysis of the small number of patients with positive pH monitoring was not done. This could be helpful in determining if a positive pH study predicted symptom response to PPI therapy.

Two additional placebo-controlled, randomized double-blinded studies primarily investigating reflux-associated laryngitis and PPIs showed no difference in laryngeal symptoms (including cough, globus, throat clearing, sore throat, and hoarseness) when treated with placebo versus PPIs.[25,26] Noordzij et al[25] found that there was no statistical improvement in cough severity when treated with omeprazole 40 mg BID compared to placebo. The cough score, however, was an average of severity and frequency among the entire study group and may not have reflected individual responses. Similarly, Havas et al[26] showed a slight improvement in an undisclosed number of patients with cough, but there was no statistical difference between the placebo group and the group of patients receiving lansoprazole 30 mg BID.

Ours et al[7] investigated the role of omeprazole 40 mg bid versus placebo in the diagnosis and treatment of chronic cough in a double-blinded, randomized, placebo-controlled design. After excluding other causes of chronic cough, 23 patients were stratified based on 24-hour pH testing and then randomized to PPI or placebo. All patients underwent pH monitoring using a dual-probe transnasal system and esophageal manometry. Symptoms were assessed using a cough frequency/severity scale at baseline, 3, 6, 9, and 12 weeks, and longer in patients who responded to PPIs. At the end of the study, randomized patients received open label PPI and continued their cough diary for an additional 4 weeks. Among the 17 patients with abnormal pH results, only six (35%) had a dramatic response to treatment. Five of these, however, received placebo initially and only improved in the one-month follow-up period with open label omperazole. This, in effect, acts as a crossover study, without concurrent placebo control or physician blinding, negating the validity of the initial double-blinded placebo-controlled design. Importantly, all six patients in the normal pH group receiving open-label omeprazole did not improve. Although flawed, this study illustrates a few important points. Patients with normal esophageal pH tests did not respond to bid PPI, corroborating the results of the Vaezi study.[12] Among patients with abnormal pH tests, only 35% improved on bid PPI. This may represent inadequate acid suppression, but more likely another etiology for the cough altogether. Follow-up pH data on PPI therapy would be helpful in determining the adequacy of acid suppression and help identify if these nonresponders truly have GERD-related cough.

With the exception of the Ours study, the remainder of the negative studies investigated improvement of reflux-associated posterior laryngopharyngitis as the primary endpoint. These studies have heterogeneous patient populations, differing inclusion criteria, and pre- and postsurgical treatment evaluation and study designs, making generalization of the combined outcomes difficult. This highlights the lack of well-designed, randomized placebo-controlled medical treatment studies primarily evaluating the role of GERD specifically in cough.

Cochrane Review

In 2006, Chang et al[37] published a systematic review and meta-analysis of randomized controlled trials of gastroesophageal reflux interventions for chronic cough associated with GERD. Using Cocharane collaboration methods and software, the authors examined 11 studies; however, the meta-analysis was limited to five studies in adults that compared PPI with placebo.[7,23,25,26,38] These studies, though randomized and controlled, have limitations already outlined in this review. The meta-analysis showed no effect in the pooled analysis of the main outcomes, although all studies favored PPI. They calculated a number needed to treat (NNT) of 5 although the confidence interval included infinity. The authors concluded that PPIs probably have some effect on GERD related cough in adults, but the effect is not universal.

Surgical Treatment Studies

All surgical treatment studies reviewed observed a marked improvement in chronic cough after fundoplication with the exception of the study by Swoger et al.[35] Most studies were cohort studies done in patients with well-documented esophageal acid reflux usually by pH testing,[27-34] but few had documented evidence of successful acid suppression prior to surgery.[35,36]

Patients with Documented GERD and Abnormal Esophageal Acid Exposure

Six prospective cohort studies examined the outcomes of surgical antireflux procedures.[27,29-33] Study sizes were variable, ranging from 24 to 324 patients. In all these studies, GERD was well defined by typical reflux symptoms, endoscopy (presence of esophagitis and/or hiatal hernia), manometry, and pH study. Various questionnaires and occasionally quality of life measurements were used for follow-up, which ranged from 12 months to 20 months (average 16.5 months, one not reported[33]). All reports found a significant improvement in cough symptoms ranging from 58% to 92%.

Although most of these cohorts compare similar patients with GERD, Farrell et al[32] divided patients into three groups based on severity of typical and atypical symptoms: Group 1 had severe typical and minimal atypical symptoms, Group 2 had both severe typical and atypical symptoms, and Group 3 had minimal typical but severe atypical symptoms. In this prospective cohort of 324 patients undergoing laparoscopic fundoplication, 97% of patients with chronic cough (67/324) had some response (~65% resolved, ~30% improvement). Response was determined by a symptom severity score (SSS) questionnaire evaluating typical and atypical symptoms (heartburn, cough, chest pain, hoarseness, asthma) administered preoperatively and at 6 and 52 weeks postoperatively. All groups had significant improvement in all symptoms (>90%); however, Group 1 had a statistically better improvement in typical symptoms than did Group 2 (99% versus 95%). Among group 3 (those with primarily atypical and few typical symptoms), 48% had resolution of symptoms whereas an additional 46% had improvement. Unfortunately, only 56 patients had cough at baseline, and the response rate was only communicated in histogram form.

Two retrospective cohort studies attempted to elicit symptom response to antireflux surgery.[28,34] Thoman et al[28] retrospectively reviewed 129 patients who underwent laparoscopic fundoplication, 37 of whom preoperatively had cough as a primary complaint. All patients had gastroesophageal reflux demonstrated by upper endoscopy or 24-hour pH monitoring. Nearly all patients had either complete resolution (65%), or significant improvement (27%) in their cough as determined by questionnaire. Greason et al[34] demonstrated a 60% improvement in cough in 65 patients who underwent a variety of surgical procedures for GERD with concurrent respiratory symptoms. A total of 30 patients had cough as a primary symptom prior to surgery. All patients had surgery primarily for GERD, though the diagnosis was determined in a variety of ways in a nonstandardized fashion: only 16 patients had pH study, 46 had esophagitis based on EGD or barium study, and typical GERD symptoms were present in 60 of 65 patients.

All of these cohort studies, both prospective and retrospective, share the same shortcomings: (1) detailed preoperative medication trials and patient response are not discussed; (2) no postoperative objective measurement of acid suppression is made (ie, no postoperative 24-hour pH monitoring) to assess the adequacy of surgery in preventing reflux; and (3) by definition, these cohort groups lack controls, questioning the validity of their outcomes. Furthermore, there is an inherent bias, especially in the surgical literature, of not reporting negative or unfavorable studies.

Patients with Normal Esophageal Acid Exposure

Unlike the studies in the previous section where the vast majority of patients have typical symptoms, erosive esophagitis, pH-defined GERD, but an unknown response to medical therapy, two studies specifically examined the role of surgery in patients with persistent chronic cough despite the normalization of pH studies by medical therapy.[35,36]

In a prospective concurrent controlled study, Swoger et al[35] compared Nissen fundoplication versus medical therapy in 25 patients with laryngeal symptoms including cough.[35] Thirty percent of patients in the surgical group and 31% in the control group had cough as a primary or secondary symptom. All patients had pH evidence of acid reflux *off* medication and symptoms were unresponsive to a four-month trial of twice-daily PPI. All patients also had baseline manometry, dual probe pH tests and Bilitec done on PPI therapy, the latter to assess bile reflux, as well as laryngoscopy. Ten patients elected to undergo Nissen fundoplication. These patients had persistent symptoms despite normalized pH *on* BID PPIs and were followed up with BRAVO capsule pH monitoring, laryngoscopy, and manometry at 3 months, and with questionnaires at 1, 2, 6, and 12 months. The control group consisted of the remaining 15 patients who continued bid PPI, and who were assessed with symptom questionnaires at 1 year. Both groups had minimal improvement in their laryngeal symptoms despite adequate acid suppression as measured by pH monitoring: 1 of 10 (10%) and 1 of 15 (7%) in the surgical and medical groups, respectively. More patients improved after initiating treatment for other potential cough etiologies: 2 of 10 (20%) in the surgical group responded to treatment for asthma and allergies, 9 of 15 (60%) in the medical group responded to alcohol cessation, asthma, and allergy treatment. The individual response in cough patients was not delineated. This again illustrates the importance of performing a comprehensive history and physical, and exploring other causes of cough in patients not responding to aggressive bid PPI therapy.

Novitsky[36] et al investigated cough response in 21 patients with "silent GERD." All patients had cough for more than 8 weeks, were unresponsive to intensive lifestyle and medical therapy, and underwent a previously described diagnostic algorithm consisting of history and physical, chest and sinus radiographs, barium esophagography, methacholine inhalation challenge, bronchoscopy, gastric emptying studies, 24-hour pH monitoring, and EGD. Dual-probe pH monitoring was performed *on* medication and cough events were recorded in a diary. A cough was considered induced by a refluxate only when it occurred simultaneously or within 3 minutes of a decrease in pH to less than 4 or an increase in pH to more than 8 (surrogate marker for alkaline reflux). Altough the total percent time of esophageal pH <4 was normal in all patients on PPI therapy, many still had some acidic reflux episodes. Only 36% of cough episodes appeared to be induced by either acidic or alkaline refluxate (17.7% and 18.5%, respectively). The authors do not comment on the proportion of cough episodes *causing* reflux, nor do they explain the etiology of the remaining 64% of cough episodes. Nevertheless, postfundoplication questionnaire at a follow-up of 6 to 12 weeks and 1 year demonstrated significantly reduced Adverse Cough Outcome Survey (ACOS) and Sickness Impact Profile (SIP). Overall, 86% of patients (18/21) had improvement in cough, 62% with complete resolution and 14% with significant improvement, and only 10% noted mild-moderate improvement. No objective postoperative data were reported.

These studies are in stark contrast to each other, and raise a perplexing question: Can gastroesophageal reflux disease cause clinically significant chronic cough despite normalized esophageal acid exposure? As discussed previously, even small amounts of esophageal acid may provoke or increase cough responsiveness to other stimuli through a vagally mediated response. This may be abolished by vagotomy during fundoplication, as vagal nerve injury defined by abnormal pancreatic polypeptide secretion in response to sham feedings after fundoplication, and has been reported in 42% of surgical patients.[39] Nonacid reflux is another possible etiology in up to 25% of patients with persistent cough despite maximal acid suppression,[18] however, multichannel intraluminal impedance(MII)-pH monitoring was not done in these two studies, and is not readily available except for selected tertiary academic centers. The small sample size of the Swoger study prevents adequate interpretation and comparison. The Novitsky study lacks objective measurements in the follow-up period. The large number of unexplained cough episodes and lack of a true cough monitor (manometry proven cough episode) bring into question the reliability of the reported reflux-cough association. Also, while the patients in the Novitsky study may serve as their own controls (failed intensive medical therapy), it is difficult to determine the effectiveness of a surgical procedure when there are no true control patients and the only surgical outcome assessment is a questionnaire.

DIAGNOSIS AND TREATMENT ALGORITHM

Several observations can be made based on the data available to date:

1. The presence of typical signs or symptoms alone do not confidently make the diagnosis of GERD-related cough given the high prevalence of both GERD and other causes of cough.
2. However, patients with signs (ie, erosive esophagitis) or classical symptoms of GERD are more likely to have improvement in cough with PPI therapy or antireflux surgery.
3. A high placebo response has been seen in studies of patients with GERD and cough, making uncontrolled studies difficult to interpret.
4. On pH testing, coughing and acid reflux may coexist. However, cough *precedes* reflux in the majority of patients, making the temporal relationship of symptoms with reflux key.
5. On PPIs, a small subset of patients may have nonacid reflux causing the cough. This diagnosis requires MII-pH testing and symptom analysis to define accurately.

Based on review of the available data, we suggest the following algorithm for the diagnosis and treatment of GERD-related cough (Fig 8–2).

Detailed and compulsive history taking and physical examination are critical first steps in the evaluation of patients with cough. Our literature review suggests acid-related cough is uncommon and most chronic coughers have multiple etiologies. Therefore, time is better spent and tests less expensive when attention is focused on the more frequent causes of cough including postnasal drip, smoking, asthma, and medications.

Once other etiologies of cough are excluded, we recommend wireless BRAVO pH monitoring be performed with the patient not taking PPIs. Compared to the transnasal pH test, this procedure allows studies in a more normal physiologic state and for prolonged periods of at least 48 hours. Studies can easily be

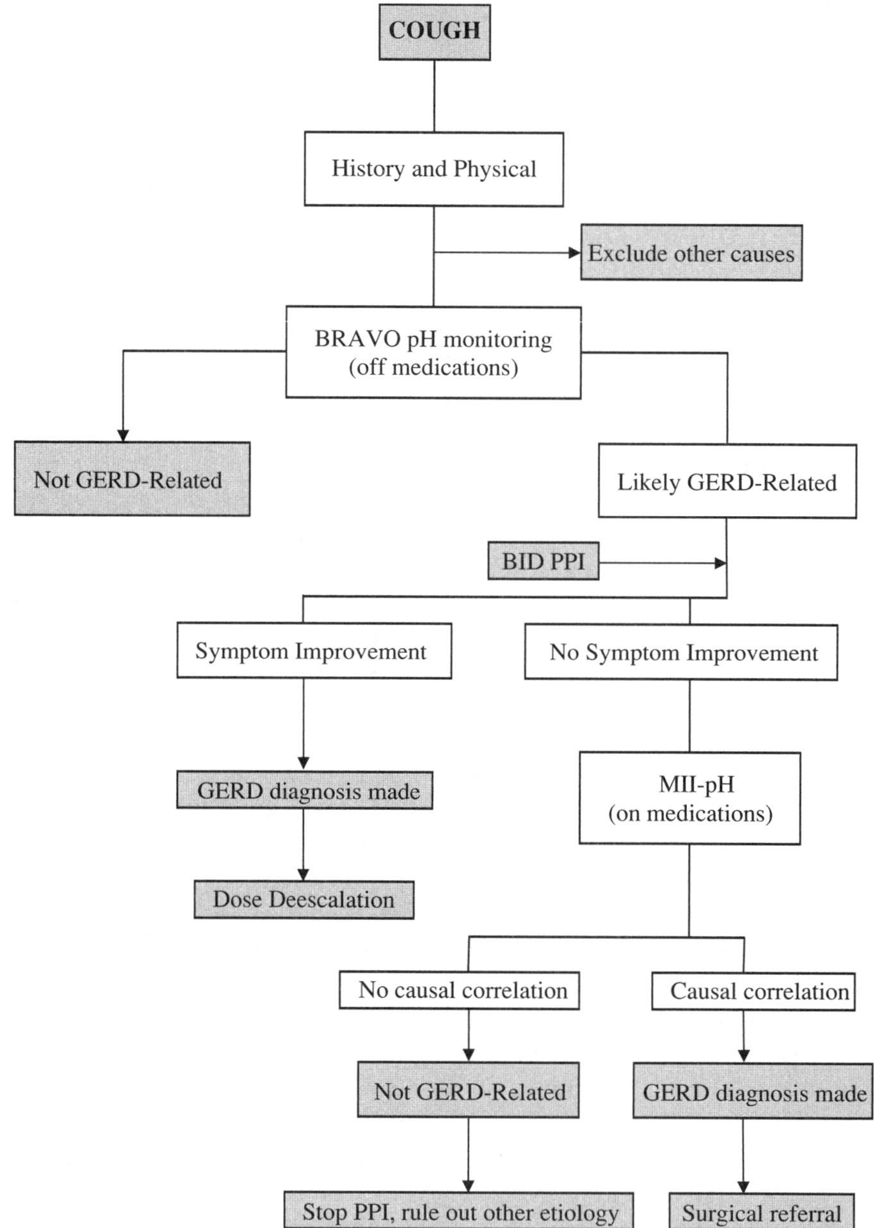

Fig 8–2. Suggested algorithm for the diagnosis and treatment of suspected GERD-related cough.

extended to 96 hours, just by having the patient return, downloading the 48 hour data, and replacing the battery.[40] Additionally, the endoscopy performed to attach the capsule adds valuable information about the presence of a hiatal hernia and esophagitis. Interpretation of BRAVO results should be made after reviewing the tracings carefully with the patient, and inquiring about the relationship between cough and meals, activities and pH drops <4. If there is no or minimal acid reflux, or if symptoms are not temporally related to reflux events, then GERD effectively can be ruled out as the etiology of cough. This avoids unneeded treatment and may facilitate the proper diagnosis by not delaying other evaluations. Although some may advocate empiric treatment with BID PPIs before pH monitoring, in reality most patients referred to gastroenterologists have already been prescribed PPIs by their primary care physicians without symptom improvement. Furthermore, the high placebo response rate seen in the patients[7,12,25,26] could lead to misdiagnosis and unnecessary PPI use for a prolonged length of time. This can be of substantial cost to the patient (generic over-the-counter omeprazole costs ~$45 per month for BID treatment) with no benefit, and again delays the proper diagnosis.

If no other cause of cough is found, and patients have significant abnormal amounts of acid reflux and/or temporally related acid reflux and coughing by pH monitoring, GERD becomes a more likely cause of cough. Medical therapy with BID PPIs taken before breakfast and dinner for 2 months should then be initiated. This regimen is extremely effective in normalizing acid reflux, with fewer than 5% of patients with extraesophageal GERD having persistent acid reflux.[21] If symptoms respond, then a gradual dose taper over months can determine the minimal amount of PPIs needed for symptom relief.

In the small number of patients with suspected GERD-related cough not responding to BID PPIs, multichannel intraluminal impedance (MII)-pH monitoring while on PPI therapy may be helpful in identifying patients with nonacid or refractory acid reflux. This technology, however, is not readily available (even at some large academic referral centers), and results should be carefully analyzed to identify the temporal relationship to symptoms ensuring that reflux is causing the cough, not vice versa. Patients with persistent cough without a temporal relationship to reflux of acid or nonacid material effectively have GERD ruled out as the cause of cough, and PPIs can be stopped for treatment of cough.

In the exceedingly small group of patients who have persistent cough that is temporally caused by acid or nonacid reflux despite maximal medical therapy, referral to a gastrointestinal surgeon for consideration of an antireflux operation is indicated. However, the patient must be cautioned that the results may not be as good as the 90% quoted for more classic reflux symptoms of heartburn and acid regurgitation.[32,41]

FUTURE DIRECTIONS

Several issues remain regarding GERD and cough including treatment of nonacid reflux, accurate temporal cough-reflux monitoring, and the need for better treatment studies.

Although Mainie has reported an excellent response of extraesophageal symptoms in patients with nonacid reflux in a small case series,[41] larger studies need to be performed to assess the effectiveness of antireflux surgery in this subset of cough patients. Other studies are also needed to better investigate medical treatments of nonacid reflux including the use of baclofen and its derivatives to impair transient LES relaxation. Possibly a good cough response to these drugs in patients with associated nonacid reflux might predict a favorable response to surgery, similar to the relationship between symptom relief of acid reflux on PPIs predicting the success of antireflux surgery.

Development and implementation of an accurate, effective cough monitor is key to accurately assessing the temporal relationship between reflux and cough. While simultaneous pH-manometry is currently the most accurate means of assessment, it is cumbersome and limited by short sampling period. The temporal relationship observed between symptoms and reflux on pH studies must be carefully reviewed and discussed with the patient to assure reliability, but still may not accurately discriminate between reflux→cough and cough→reflux.

As discussed in this review, the current literature pertaining to GERD and cough is lacking well-designed, large, randomized placebo-controlled studies evaluating the efficacy of medical and surgical management of suspected GERD-related cough. A valuable study would be one in which a large numbers of PPI naïve patients with chronic cough are followed from presentation through the algorithm detailed in Figure 8-3, following similar guidelines as described above. This approach de-emphasizes the response to PPI as the diagnostic standard, but rather utilizes temporally and symptomatically related pH data for diagnosis. The effectiveness of medications versus placebo in relieving symptoms would be more accurately evaluated in patients with well-defined GERD. This strategy would also give a more accurate estimate of the true prevalence of GERD as a cause of cough, and effectively evaluate the placebo response in patients with a high likelihood of GERD-related cough.

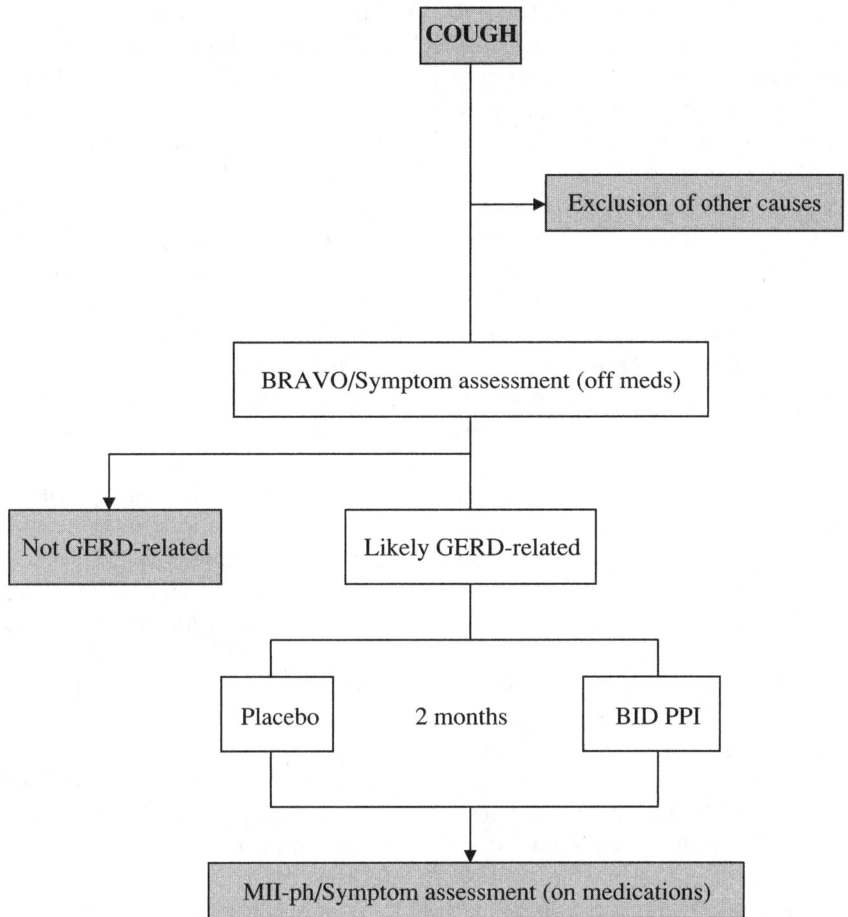

Fig 8–3. Outline of potential study to assess the role of PPI's in suspected GERD-related cough. This trial would take advantage of the new available tests to better measure acid- and nonacid GER.

REFERENCES

1. Jaspersen D, Kulig M, Labenz J, et al. Prevalence of extra-oesophageal manifestations in gastro-oesophageal reflux disease: an analysis based on the ProGERD Study. *Aliment Pharmacol Ther.* 2003; 17(12):1515–1520.
2. Locke GR 3rd, Talley NJ, Fett SL, et al. Prevalence and clinical spectrum of gastroesophageal reflux: a population-based study in Olmsted County, Minnesota. *Gastroenterology.* 1997;112(5): 1448–1456.
3. Holmes RL, Fadden CT. Evaluation of the patient with chronic cough. *Am Fam Physician.* 2004;69(9):2159–2166.
4. Hing E, Cherry DK, Woodwell DA. National Ambulatory Health Care Survey: 2004 summary. *Advance Data from Vital and Health Statistics*, Vol 374, Hyattsville, MD: National Center for Health Statistics; 2006.

5. Irwin RS, Curley FJ, French CL. Chronic cough. The spectrum and frequency of causes, key components of the diagnostic evaluation, and outcome of specific therapy. *Am Rev Respir Dis.* 1990;141(3): 640-647.
6. French, CL, Irwin RS, Curley FJ, Krikorian CJ. Impact of chronic cough on quality of life. *Arch Int Med.* 1998;158(15): 1657-1661.
7. Ours TM, Kavuru MS, Schilz RJ, et al. A prospective evaluation of esophageal testing and a double-blind, randomized study of omeprazole in a diagnostic and therapeutic algorithm for chronic cough. *Am J Gastroenterol.* 1999;94(11): 3131-3138.
8. Canning BJ. Anatomy and neurophysiology of the cough reflex: ACCP evidence-based clinical practice guidelines. *Chest.* 2006;129(1 suppl):33S-47S.
9. Canning BJ, Mazzone SB. Reflex mechanisms in gastroesophageal reflux disease and asthma. *Am J Med.* 2003;115(suppl 3A):45S-48S.
10. Ing AJ, Ngu MC, Breslin AB. Pathogenesis of chronic persistent cough associated with gastroesophageal reflux. *Am J Respir Crit Care Med.* 1994;149(1):160-167.
11. Wu DN, Yamauchi K, Kobayashi H, et al. Effects of esophageal acid perfusion on cough responsiveness in patients with bronchial asthma. *Chest.* 2002;122(2): 505-509.
12. Vaezi MF, Richter JE, Stasney CR, et al. Treatment of chronic posterior laryngitis with esomeprazole. *Laryngoscope.* 2006; 116(2):254-260.
13. Poelmans J, Feenstra L, Demedts I, et al. The yield of upper gastrointestinal endoscopy in patients with suspected reflux-related chronic ear, nose, and throat symptoms. *Am J Gastroenterol.* 2004; 99(8):1419-1426.
14. Pandolfino JE, Richter JE, Ours T, et al. Ambulatory esophageal pH monitoring using a wireless system. *Am J Gastroenterol.* 2003;98(4):740-749.
15. Irwin RS, French CL, Curley FJ, et al. Chronic cough due to gastroesophageal reflux. Clinical, diagnostic, and pathogenetic aspects. *Chest.* 1993;104(5):1511-1517.
16. Zerbib F, Roman S, Ropert A, et al. Esophageal pH-impedance monitoring and symptom analysis in GERD: a study in patients off and on therapy. *Am J Gastroenterol.* 2006;101(9):1956-1963.
17. Sifrim D, Dupont L, Blondeau K, et al. Weakly acidic reflux in patients with chronic unexplained cough during 24 hour pressure, pH, and impedance monitoring. *Gut.* 2005;54(4):449-454.
18. Tutuian R, Mainie I, Agrawal A, et al. Nonacid reflux in patients with chronic cough on acid-suppressive therapy. *Chest.* 2006;130(2):386-391.
19. Johnston BT, Troshinsky MB, Castell JA, et al. Comparison of barium radiology with esophageal pH monitoring in the diagnosis of gastroesophageal reflux disease. *Am J Gastroenterol.* 1996;91(6): 1181-1185.
20. Barnes TW, Afessa B, Swanson KL, et al. The clinical utility of flexible bronchoscopy in the evaluation of chronic cough. *Chest.* 2004;126(1):268-272.
21. Vaezi MF, Schroeder PL, Richter JE. Reproducibility of proximal probe pH parameters in 24-hour ambulatory esophageal pH monitoring. *Am J Gastroenterol.* 1997;92(5):825-829.
22. Baldi F, Cappiello R, Cavoli C, et al. Proton pump inhibitor treatment of patients with gastroesophageal reflux-related chronic cough: a comparison between two different daily doses of lansoprazole. *World J Gastroenterol.* 2006;12(1):82-88.
23. Kiljander TO, Salomaa ER, Hietanen EK, et al. Chronic cough and gastro-oesophageal reflux: a double-blind placebo-controlled study with omeprazole. *Eur Respir J.* 2000;16(4):633-638.
24. Dore MP, Pedroni A, Pes GM, et al. Effect of antisecretory therapy on atypical symptoms in gastroesophageal reflux disease. *Dig Dis Sci.* 2007;52(2):463-468.

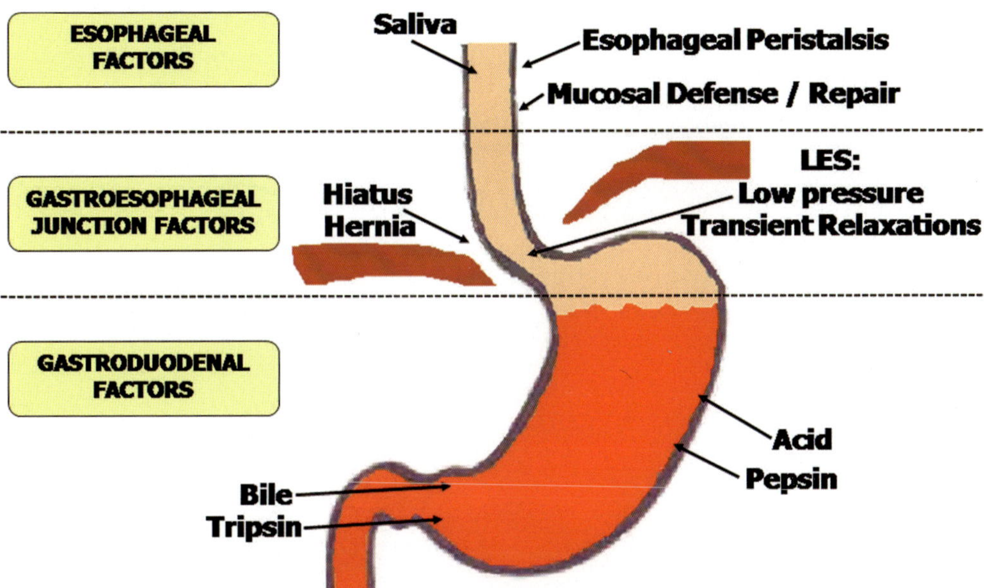

Color Plate 1. Factors contributing to gastroesophageal reflux and esophageal injury. Reflux of gastric contents into the esophagus occurs as a result of the interplay among different factors in the upper gastrointestinal tract. Potentially harmful agents to the esophageal mucosa or supraesophageal structures include gastric acid and pepsin, as well as duodenal secretions including bile and trypsin. The lower esophageal sphincter (LES), in concert with the crural diaphragm forms a barrier at the gastroesophageal junction in order to prevent movement of harmful gastroduodenal contents into the esophagus. This barrier may be breached during transient lower esophageal relaxations, or due to a hypotensive LES or other mechanisms associated with the presence of a hiatal hernia. Once esophageal mucosa is exposed to the damaging gastroduodenal agents, luminal protection occurs through esophageal clearance of refluxate (peristalsis), acid neutralization by saliva, and epithelial defense and repair mechanisms. When the esophagogastric junction is breached with enough frequency to overwhelm the esophageal or supraesophageal protective mechanisms, symptoms and injury may develop.

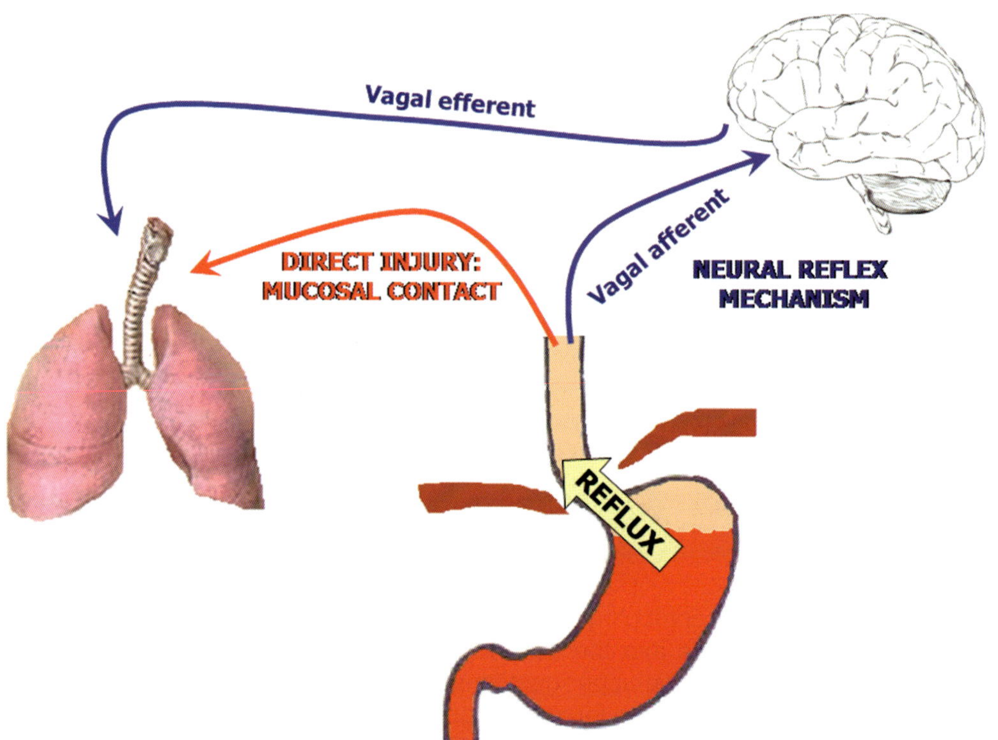

Color Plate 2. Mechanisms of extraesophageal damage due to gastroesophageal reflux. Gastroesophageal reflux may lead to pulmonary and laryngeal complications by two separate mechanisms. Reflux may extend proximally beyond the esophagus, damaging supraesophageal structures through direct injury as a consequence of mucosal contact (*shown in red*). Pulmonary and laryngeal disease may also be triggered by a vagally mediated neural reflex pathway (*shown in blue*), whereby presence of refluxate in the esophagus stimulates vagal afferents, with subsequent efferent signals causing changes in the lung and larynx, such as bronchoconstriction or glottal closure.

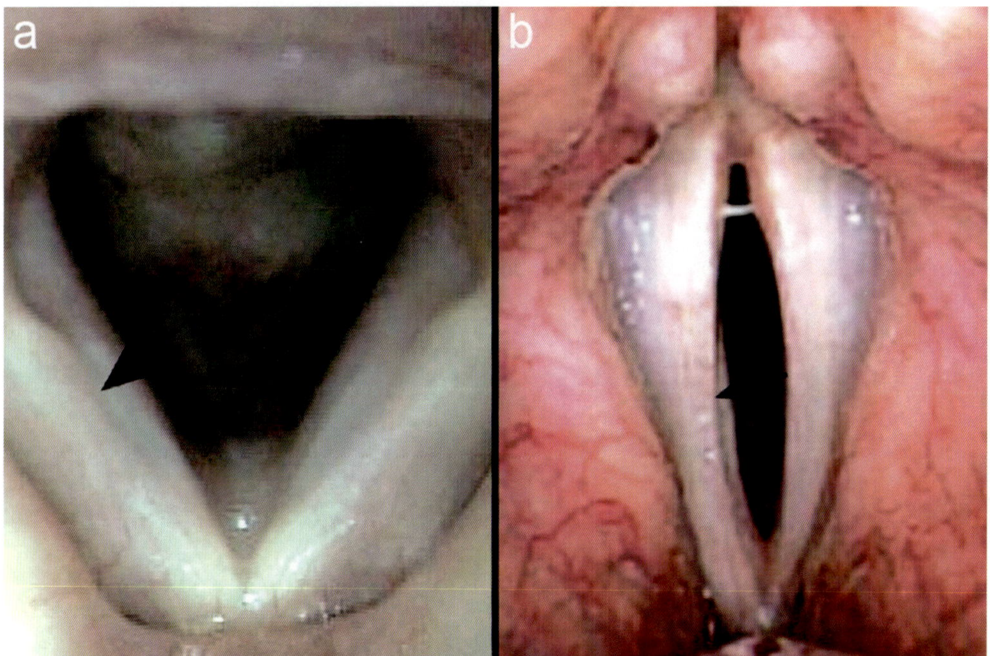

Color Plate 3. Pseudosulcus vocalis versus sulcus vocalis. **A.** In pseudosulcus vocalis, diffuse edema is present along the entire length of the vocal fold and extends to the subglottis. This creates the appearance of an indentation within the vocal fold (*left arrow*). **B.** Conversely, in sulcus vocalis, loss of the lamina propria causes a true indendation within the true vocal fold itself. Reproduced with permission from Belafsky PC, Postma GN, Koufman JA. The validity and reliability of the reflux finding score (RFS). *Laryngoscope.* 2001;111(8):1313–1317. Copyright 2001 by Lippincott-Williams & Wilkins.

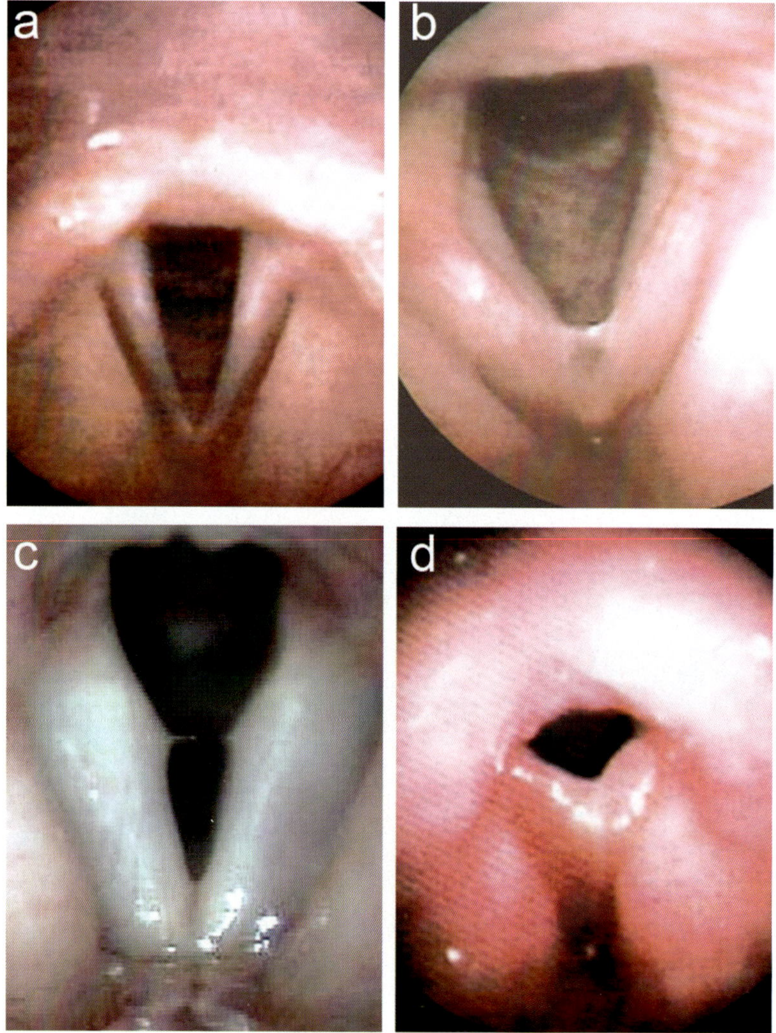

Color Plate 4. Endoscopic findings consistent with LPR. **A.** Normal larynx with no posterior commisure hypertrophy, open ventricular space, and no laryngeal edema. **B.** Moderate posterior commisure hypertrophy, moderate vocal fold edema, subglottic edema with pseudosulcus vocalis, partial ventricular obliteration, and diffuse laryngeal edema. **C.** Diffuse edema causing obliteration of the ventricular space, severe true vocal fold edema, and mild posterior commisure hypertrophy. **D.** Severe true and false vocal fold edema with polypoid degeneration of the true vocal fold, severe posterior commisure hypertrophy, diffuse erythema, and obliteration of the ventricle. Reproduced with permission from Belafsky PC, Postma GN, Koufman JA. The validity and reliability of the reflux finding score (RFS). *Laryngoscope.* 2001;111(8):1313–1317. Copyright 2001 by Lippincott-Williams & Wilkins.

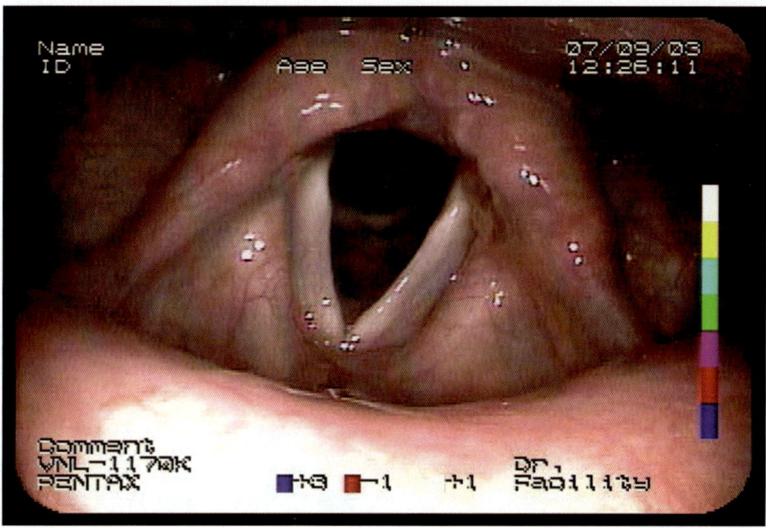

Color Plate 5. Larynx showing posterior glottic edema, obliteration of ventricles, and vocal fold edema.

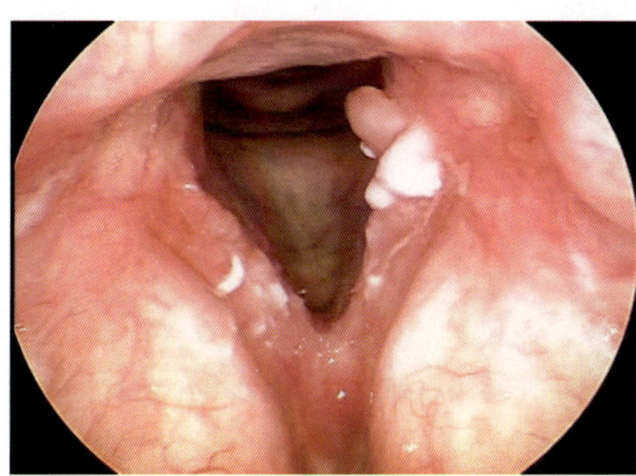

Color Plate 6. Larynx showing a protruding vocal process granuloma. Note the excess mucus on and around the vocal folds and the abnormal condition of the vocal folds.

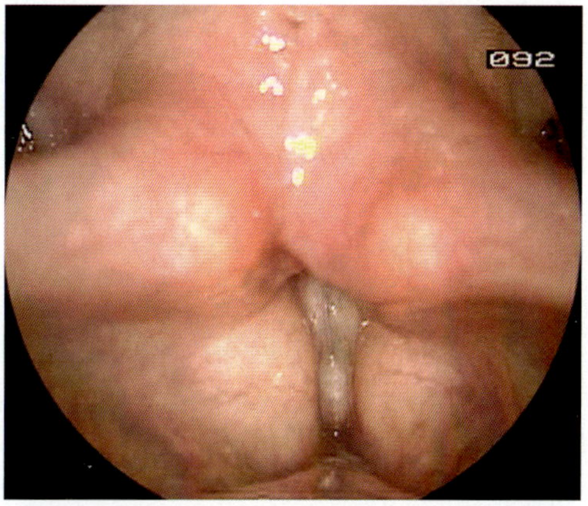

Color Plate 7. Supraglottic hyperfunction consistent with MTD.

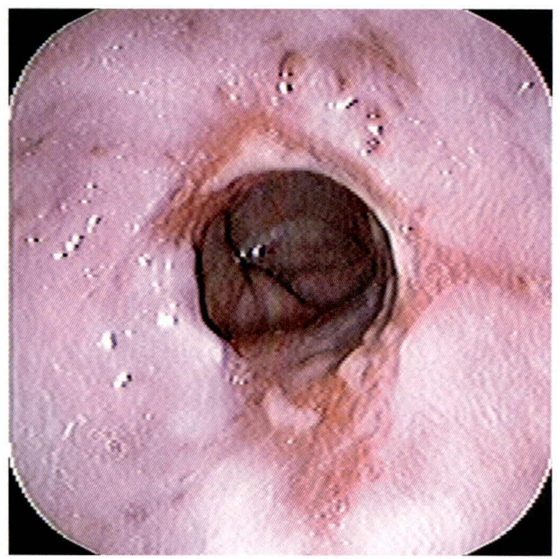

Color Plate 8. Distal esophageal peptic stricture with erosive esophagitis and hiatal hernia.

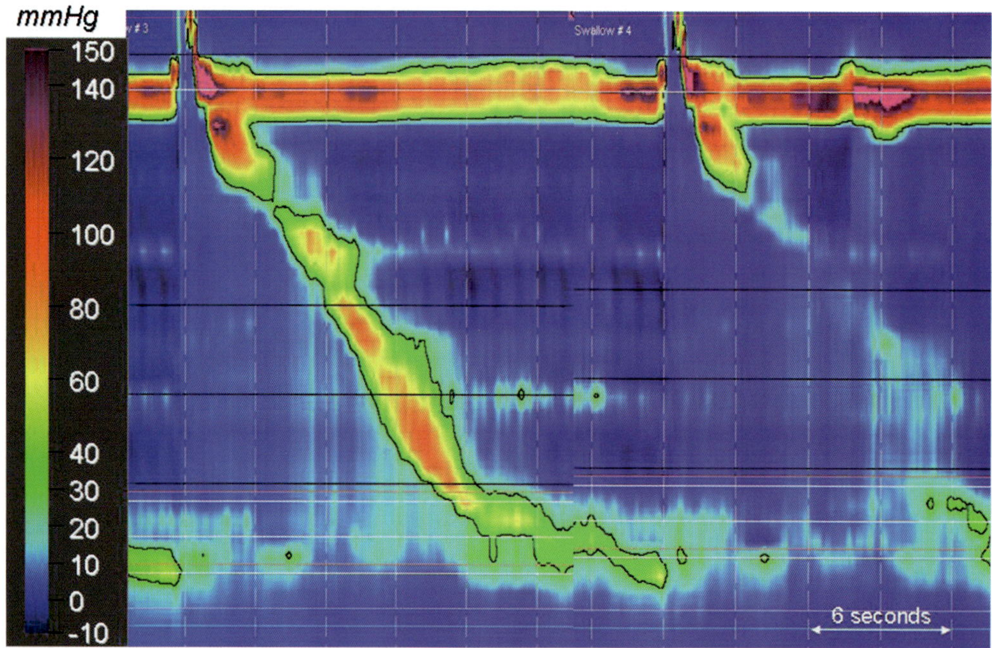

Color Plate 9. High-resolution esophageal manometry contour plot recording from a patient with GERD depicting a normal peristaltic sequence followed by a failed or ineffective water swallow. The horizontal, red band at the top of the plot represents the upper esophageal sphincter whereas the lower, green region is the lower esophageal sphincter with periods of deglutitive relaxation. The diagonal propagating front seen with the first swallow sequence is a normal peristaltic contraction. This is notably absent in the second, failed swallow although lower esophageal sphincter relaxation is observed. The isobaric contour in this plot is set at 30 mm Hg such that all pressures of 30 mm Hg are outlined in black.

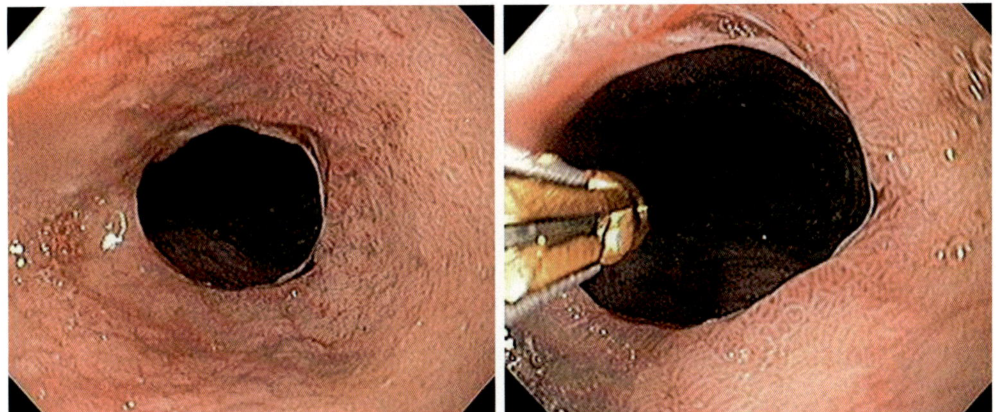

Color Plate 10. Large, circumferential esophageal inlet patch with cervical esophageal stricture at distal aspect of patch.

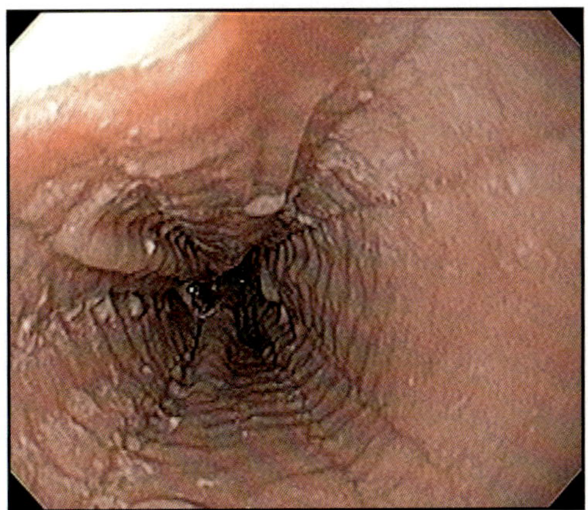

Color Plate 11. Eosinophilic esophagitis with mucosal rings, fine-reticular exudates, and longitudinal furrows.

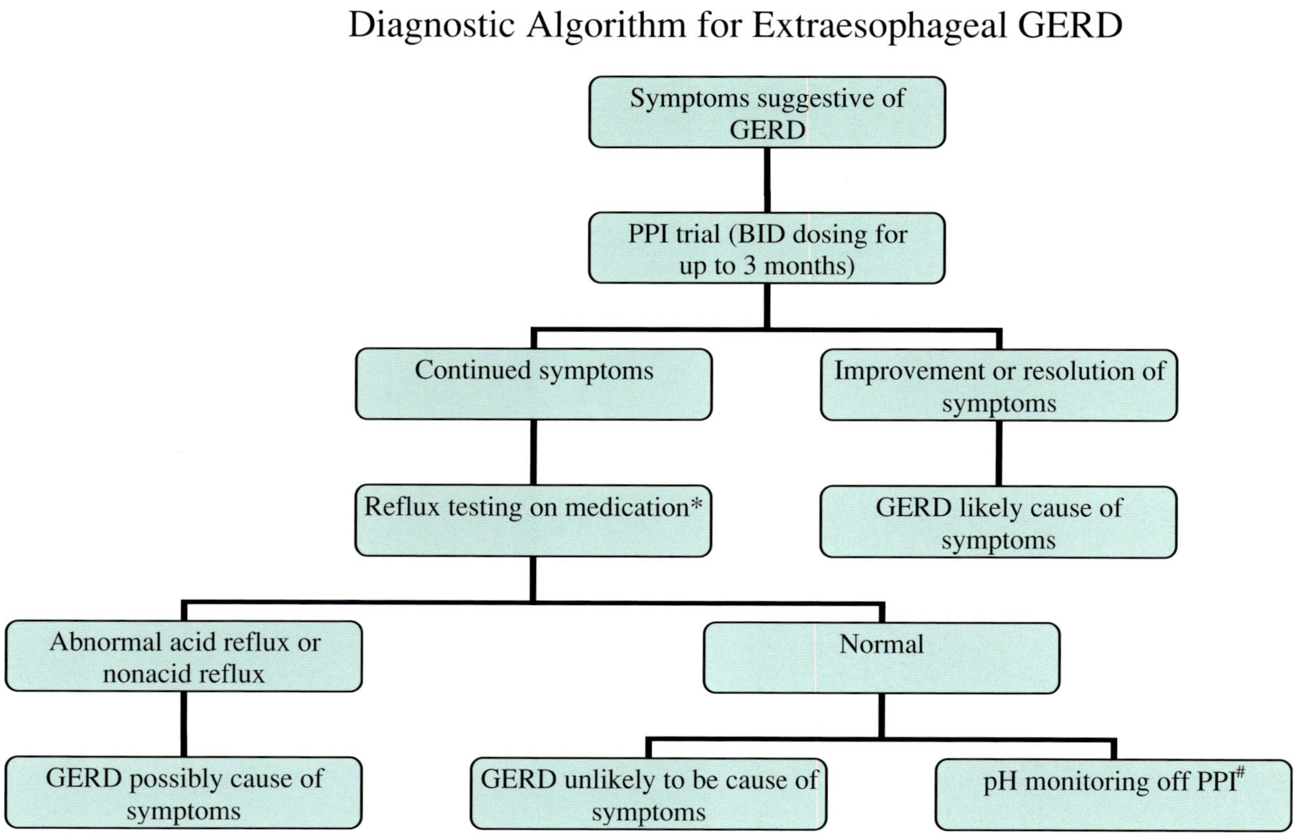

*Combined pH and impedance monitoring or 48-hour Bravo monitoring

#To determine if reflux is present though not necessarily related

Color Plate 12. Diagnostic algorithm for extraesophageal GERD.

25. Noordzij JP, Khidr A, Evans BA, et al. Evaluation of omeprazole in the treatment of reflux laryngitis: a prospective, placebo-controlled, randomized, double-blind study. *Laryngoscope.* 2001;111(12):2147-2151.
26. Havas TO, Huang S, Levy M, et al. Posterior pharyngolaryngitis: double-blind randomised placebo-controlled trial of proton pump inhibitor therapy. *Austr J Otolaryngol.* 1999;3:243-246.
27. Ekström T, Johansson KE. Effects of anti-reflux surgery on chronic cough and asthma in patients with gastro-oesophageal reflux disease. *Respir Med.* 2000;94(12):1166-1167.
28. Thoman DS, Hui TT, Spyrou M, et al. Laparoscopic antireflux surgery and its effect on cough in patients with gastroesophageal reflux disease. *J Gastrointest Surg.* 2002;6(1):17-21.
29. Brouwer R, Kiroff GK. Improvement of respiratory symptoms following laparoscopic Nissen fundoplication. *ANZ J Surg.* 2003;73(4):189-193.
30. Wright RC, Rhodes KP. Improvement of laryngopharyngeal reflux symptoms after laparoscopic Hill repair. *Am J Surg.* 2003;185(5):455-461.
31. Duffy JP, Maggard M, Hiyama DT, et al. Laparoscopic Nissen fundoplication improves quality of life in patients with atypical symptoms of gastroesophageal reflux. *Am Surg.* 2003;69(10):833-838.
32. Farrell TM, Richardson WS, Trus TL, et al. Response of atypical symptoms of gastro-oesophageal reflux to antireflux surgery. *Br J Surg.* 2001;88(12):1649-1652.
33. Rakita S, Villadolid D, Thomas A, et al. Laparoscopic Nissen fundoplication offers high patient satisfaction with relief of extraesophageal symptoms of gastroesophageal reflux disease. *Am Surg.* 2006;72(3):207-212.
34. Greason KL, Miller DL, Deschamps C, et al. Effects of antireflux procedures on respiratory symptoms. *Ann Thorac Surg.* 2002;73(2):381-385.
35. Swoger J, Ponsky J, Hicks DM, et al. Surgical fundoplication in laryngopharyngeal reflux unresponsive to aggressive acid suppression: a controlled study. *Clin Gastroenterol Hepatol.* 2006;4(4):433-441.
36. Novitsky YW, Zawacki JK, Irwin RS, et al. Chronic cough due to gastroesophageal reflux disease: efficacy of antireflux surgery. *Surg Endosc.* 2002;16(4):567-571.
37. Chang AB, Lasserson TJ, Kiljander TO, et al. Systematic review and meta-analysis of randomised controlled trials of gastro-oesophageal reflux interventions for chronic cough associated with gastro-oesophageal reflux. *Br Med J.* 2006;332(7532):11-17.
38. Eherer AJ, Habermann W, Hammer HF, et al. Effect of pantoprazole on the course of reflux-associated laryngitis: a placebo-controlled double-blind crossover study. *Scand J Gastroenterol.* 2003;38(5):462-467.
39. DeVault KR, Swain JM, Wentling GK, et al. Evaluation of vagus nerve function before and after antireflux surgery. *J Gastrointest Surg.* 2004;8(7):883-888; discussion 888-889.
40. Hirano I, Zhang Q, Pandolfino JE, et al. Four-day Bravo pH capsule monitoring with and without proton pump inhibitor therapy. *Clin Gastroenterol Hepatol.* 2005;3(11):1083-1088.
41. Mainie I, Tutuian R, Agrawal A, et al. Combined multichannel intraluminal impedance-pH monitoring to select patients with persistent gastro-oesophageal reflux for laparoscopic Nissen fundoplication. *Br J Surg.* 2006;93(12):1483-1487.

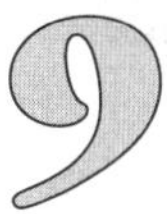

Extraesophageal Reflux: The Sinonasal Passages and Middle Ear

John W. Alldredge and Donald C. Lanza

INTRODUCTION

Sinusitis, otitis media, and gastroesophageal reflux disease (GERD) are each common disorders. Although each can present independently, some of these disorders can be important comorbidities for one another. When they are present simultaneously in a given individual, it can be very difficult to determine the role that each disorder has on the patient's quality of life or disease state. This is partly true because certain hallmark symptoms might be absent, subtle or overlapping and because there are limitations in detecting gastric reflux. To this point, 48-hour Bravo pH probe evaluations distinguish patients with GERD with a sensitivity of only 65% but a specificity of 95%.[1] Limitations in detecting gastric reflux affecting the uppermost airway has to do with many factors but might exist simply because damaging reflux occurs less frequently than every 48 hours or may only be associated with specific meal content or size. Again the signs and symptoms of reflux can also be nonspecific and vary depending on the end organ(s) involved (Table 9-1). Naturally, these circumstances have lead to diversity of opinion among clinicians (within and across specialties) as to when gastric reflux might be participating in respiratory epithelial inflammation. Despite this, evidence that specifically supports a relationship between extraesophageal reflux (EER) and inflammation of the nasal passages and even the middle ear is growing.

As previously mentioned in this textbook, laryngopharyngeal reflux (LPR), a form of EER, is the retrograde flow of gastric contents above the upper esophageal sphincter. It is differentiated clinically from GERD, where the primary site of irritation is the esophagus. Occasionally, when gastric material involves the sinonasal passages it has been referred to as supraglottic reflux or nasopharyngeal reflux (NPR). Interestingly, about 10% of

Table 9–1. Symptoms Associated with EER

Laryngeal/Pharyngeal Symptoms	Oral Cavity Symptoms
Unexplained hoarseness	Frequent unexplained thrush
Chronic throat clearing	Bitter/sour taste in mouth
Tightness in throat upon swallowing (globus)	Halitosis
Sensation of foreign body or lump in throat (globus)	Recurrent unexplained aphthous ulcers
Sensation of food getting stuck upon swallowing and need for double swallow (without regurgitation)	Unexplained angular chelitis
Unexplained soreness/achiness of anterior neck at level at or above thyroid cartilage especially during swallowing	Excessive salivation (Water brash)
Unexplained voice fatigue	Frequent sore throat
"Water brash" (reflex salivation)	**Pulmonary Symptoms**
Frequent belching	Unexplained cough—especially but limited to postprandial cough or nighttime cough
Recurring sore throat	Wheeze
	Chest tightness
	Intermittent "Burning in wind pipe"
Sinus and Nasal Symptoms	**Ear Symptoms**
Postnasal drip (typically clear)	Aural fullness, pain, pressure, clogged sensation, popping, or clicking
Nasal congestion, blockage	Adult serous middle ear fluid otherwise unexplained
Soreness described in back of nose/above soft palate	
Recurring cycle of sinus infections starting with clear postnasal drip/sore throat not associated with virus	
Detecting foul odor not otherwise explained	

all patients presenting to an otolaryngologist's office, and up to 50% of patients with hoarseness may have EER as a significant component of their underlying condition.[2]

The goal of this chapter is to summarize the concepts and evidence supporting the role of EER in supraglottic symptoms and disease involving ciliated respiratory epithelium of the sinuses. In addition, this chapter review discusses middle ear disease and EER. Prior to summarizing the data demonstrating these relationships, it is important to briefly review relevant physiology, define sinusitis, and to discuss its pathophysiology and treatment. We hope this approach will clarify the issues confronting clinicians and researchers treating reflux and sinusitis and/or otitis media.

RELATED RESPIRATORY AND UPPER DIGESTIVE TRACT PHYSIOLOGY

Somewhat surprisingly, normal sinonasal physiology and that of the upper gastrointestinal tract are more interrelated than might be expected. In fact, there are several mechanisms whereby airway disease and its treatments can alter this association. Two important relationships to keep in mind for this discussion are (1) the distribution of the autonomic nervous system to the respiratory tree and to the gastrointestinal tract and (2) the close relationship of the nasal passages to the pulmonary tree. Differences between esophageal epithelium and ciliated respiratory epithelium and the factors associated with the reflux, sinusitis and middle ear infection are also important.

The sympathetic and parasympathetic nervous systems help regulate blood flow and ongoing mucus production from the sinonasal passages as well as the gut. Both blood flow and mucus production are important to critical nasal airway functions such as airway filtration, humidification, and temperature regulation. It is estimated that the sinonasal passages produce approximately 1 liter of mucus daily to help with these functions. Typically this mucous drainage is imperceptibly swallowed. Additionally, the sinonasal airway has an important role in olfaction as well as in immune surveillance and airway protection (eg, sneeze reflex). The ciliated respiratory epithelium not only produces a mucociliary blanket which helps with filtration, humidification and temperature control but also secretes certain chemicals into this mucus called cationic antimicrobial peptides (eg, defensins) that kill inhaled bacteria, viruses, and fungi. Thus, mucociliary clearance is an essential defense mechanism against microorganisms and particulate matter. The normal pH range of the mucous is approximately 7.0 to 9.0.[3,4]

Importantly, experimental evidence suggests that the most critical role of the nasal airway is to aid in pulmonary function through *impedance matching* of the lungs to the outer environment.[5] The nasal airway supplies the appropriate amount of resistance for optimal diaphragmatic muscle contraction during normal inspiration.[5] This explains, in part, why most people preferentially breathe through their nose and not their mouth. To a point, the resistance of nasal airflow supplies tension to the muscles of the diaphragm, thereby improving the effectiveness of diaphragmatic contraction. This helps properly ventilate the lungs during normal quiet breathing. The nasal resistance also helps to regulate the rate of expiration, thus controlling oxygenation and CO_2 levels.

Through the impedance matching relationship, increases in nasal resistance, like those occurring during viral upper respiratory tract infection, seasonal allergy, or sinusitis will tend to increase the force of contraction of the diaphragm to overcome the nasal blockage in quiet breathing. This, in turn, may increase intra-abdominal pressures. Because of the external force exerted on the stomach and negative pressure generated within the pharynx, increased nasal resistance will tend to allow stomach contents to ascend the esophagus. This is believed to be more common in obstructive sleep apnea where negative pressures are most extreme and where reflux is more likely in the supine position during sleep.[5-7]

The frequency and severity of gastric reflux is dependent on many factors.

Important factors associated with gastric reflux include: the volume of stomach contents (increased acid production), gastric motility and emptying, and the effectiveness of the upper and lower esophageal sphincters (LES). This includes the relationship to the diaphragm. Additionally, diet, food supplements, medications, gastric contents near the LES (eg, hiatal hernia, supine position, bending), weakness of the diaphragmatic crural muscle, and increased intra-abdominal pressure as with pregnancy, obesity, and forceful coughing are all important variables promoting reflux.[8] Traditionally, a measured pH below 4 is considered abnormal when evaluating for acid reflux. However, this is not believed the most accurate measurement of reflux in the more proximal pharynx, where mucosal protection is minimal.[9] Interestingly, it has been noted that pepsin retains greater than 30% of its activity at a pH of 5; moreover, the enzyme may still remain stable at pH levels up to 7.[10-12] Dobhan and Castell[13] thus have suggested that pH values less than or equal to 5 may provide a better endpoint when evaluating for reflux in the more proximal pharyngeal tissues.

The underlying pathophysiologic mechanisms of sinusitis are not completely understood. It is typically thought to begin with edema of the nasal and sinus mucosa, leading to disruption of mucociliary clearance and perhaps innate immunity (cationic antimicrobial peptides). This, in turn, can lead to inflammation, sinus obstruction, mucous stasis, ciliary dysfunction, and possible chronic infection with bacteria or fungus. There can be multiple causes of this initial inflammatory insult. These may include viral infection, bacteria, fungi, dental infection, environmental irritants, inhalant allergy, food allergy, aspirin sensitivity, immunodeficiency, cystic fibrosis, primary ciliary dyskinesia, osteitis, biofilm formation, and anatomic variation.[14]

The exact mechanism by which gastric reflux affects the paranasal sinuses is unknown; however, three theories have been proposed. The first involves a direct effect of acid or pepsin on the sinonasal mucosa. Due to the nature of the differences in epithelium and their protective barriers, it is thought that respiratory epithelial surface are more sensitive to acid induced damage that their lower esophageal counterparts.[15,16] The combination of acid exposure along with activated pepsin may cause swelling and edema, leading to impaired mucociliary function, obstruction of the sinus openings, and secondary infection. Koufman[2] demonstrated a synergistic effect of acid and pepsin in canine larynges as compared to controls where acid only was used. The second possible mechanism may involve a vagally mediated neurogenic mechanism. A dysfunctional autonomic nervous system may lead to sinonasal edema and ostial obstruction.[17] Exaggerated vagal responsiveness in the lower airways has been demonstrated in patients with asthma and GER[18,19] whereas autonomic dysfunction has also been noted in patients with chronic rhinitis and upper airway inflammation.[20] The third possible mechanism relates to the role of *Helicobacter pylori*. *H. pylori* is a gram-negative organism that has been linked to gastric ulcers and gastritis.[21] Ozdek et al[22] found evidence of *H. pylori* DNA in 4 of 12 patients using PCR techniques. Three of these four patients had complaints consistent with GER. Although intriguing, the significance of these findings is not known. In the proper clinical setting pepsin, *Helicobacter pylori*, or bilious material can be potential sources of tissue injury and inflammation, but the general consensus is that respiratory epithelium damage is more likely to be mediated by the proteolytic activity of pepsin in combination with acid than *H. pylori* infection.[23,24]

The mechanism for varying forms of middle ear infection is not completely understood, nor is the nature of NPR involvement. There are many risk factors implicated in the development of recurrent acute otitis media that include: age of child, immaturity of eustachian tube function, child daycare, season, lack of breast feeding for (conveyed immunity), adenoidal disease, second-hand smoke, pacifier use, allergy, genetic predisposition, craniofacial abnormality, and birth order.[25] Radiographic studies have shown that swallowing can bring about movement of fluid from nasopharynx into the middle ear.[26] Secondary swelling in the eustachian tube can lead to negative pressure in the middle ear. Sustained negative pressure in the middle ear has been shown to bring about middle ear effusion.[27]

RHINOSINUSITIS

Generally speaking, "sinusitis" is defined as an inflammation of the mucosa of the nasal cavity and paranasal sinuses. In and of itself the term "sinusitis" does not specify disease etiology or pathophysiology. It describes a disease state. Therefore, it is better thought of as a syndrome or a constellation of symptoms and signs. In terms of accuracy, however, the term "rhinosinusitis," rather than "sinusitis" is recommended, as sinusitis is often preceded by, and rarely occurs without, concurrent rhinitis.[28,29]

Rhinosinusitis (RS) is subdivided into several different categories based on clinical presentation. These include: acute RS, subacute RS, chronic RS (with and without polyps), recurrent acute RS, acute exacerbation of chronic RS, and fungal RS.[14,28-30] *Acute* rhinosinusitis is defined as being sudden onset, again typically preceded by viral illness and lasts up to 4 weeks in duration. *Chronic* rhinosinusitis, which may be present *with or without polyps*, is diagnosed after symptoms and or signs have been present for more 12 weeks in duration. Symptoms are usually less severe than acute, and fever is not considered a major diagnostic factor.[28] Health experts estimate 37 million Americans are affected by rhinosinusitis each year. Nearly 32 million cases of chronic sinusitis are reported to the Centers for Disease Control and Prevention annually. As such, chronic rhinosinusitis (CRS) is one of the most common chronic health conditions in the United States.[30-34]

There are many signs and symptoms associated with the diagnosis of rhinosinusitis but few are truly disease specific (Table 9-2). This may help explain why studies have shown that as many as 40% of patients referred to tertiary care rhinology clinics for evaluation and treatment of CRS, are diagnosed with disorders other than CRS. These mainly include various forms of allergic and nonallergic rhinitis, headache, facial pain, and reflux laryngitis.[35] Should the patient lack traditional symptoms associated with GERD such as heartburn, regurgitation, or even water brash (the reflex salivary hypersecretion secondary to peptic esophageal irritation) the association with rhinosinusitis is even harder to establish on the basis of history. Patients with CRS typically present with postnasal drip

Table 9–2. Symptoms and Signs Associated with Rhinosinusitis

Major Symptoms and Signs	Minor Symptoms and Signs
Facial pressure/pain	Headache (typically acute)
Facial congestion/fullness	Fever (all nonacute)
Nasal obstruction/blockage	Halitosis
Nasal discharge/purulence/ postnasal drainage	Fatigue
Hyposmia/anosmia	Dental pain
Purulence seen in nasal airway	Cough
Fever (typically in acute)	Ear pain/pressure/fullness

(PND) being a significant complaint. Wise et al[9] found that patients with NPR and LPR exhibited significantly more episodes of PND symptomatology than those without reflux. Patients may also have the previously described symptoms of LPR. Actual physical findings of reflux related CRS may include previously described findings of LPR, in addition to atrophic posterior pharyngeal mucosa, and variable amounts of erythema and edema of the nasopharynx. Importantly, comprehensive nasal and laryngeal office endoscopy can be an essential part of the complete evaluation of patients with chronic nasal symptoms.

Many of the medications used to treat the common cold, rhinosinusitis, inhalant allergy, and asthma promote EER in predisposed individuals (Table 9-3). This untoward effect confounds the determination as to whether or not EER is a primary aspect of the underlying condition or if it is the result of treatments used to alleviate respiratory disease. Regardless of cause, once EER participates in the respiratory disease ongoing damage from acid many require treatment directed at gastric acid production. Additional medications and foods that are associated with reflux are listed in Table 9-4.

Table 9–3. Pharmaceuticals for Respiratory Disorders That Potentiate Reflux

Antihistamines secondary to anticholinergic properties (Diphenhyrdamine, Benadryl®)
Decongestant (pseudoephedrine)
Expectorant/Mucous thinner (Guaifenesin, Mucinex®)
β-2 adrenergic agonists (eg, Albuterol)
Xanthines (caffeine, theophylline)
Oral steroids
Antibiotics (Amoxicillin/clavulanate, tetracycline, clindamycin)

Acute bacterial rhinosinusitis is typically differentiated from common viral upper respiratory infection based on severity of symptoms and clinical course, as the former usually requires treatment with oral antibiotics, and the latter, is treated with conservative supportive treatment such as oral analgesics, decongestants, and hydration. The enormity of OTC product line usage is delineated by

Table 9–4. Other Medications and Foods Associated with GERD

Medications	Substances/Foods/Supplements
α-Adrenergic blocker – for HTN, BPH	Nicotine
Calcium channel blockers	Alcoholic beverages
Aspirin and other NSAIDs	Fatty foods and fried foods
Quinidine	High-dose fat soluble vitamins A and E
Potassium and iron supplements	High-dose fish oil
Alendronate (Fosamax®)	Vitamin C
Nitrates—including in preserved meats	Chocolate
Sildenafil (Viagra®)	Mint
Sedatives such as diazepam (Valium®)	Caffeinated beverage (tea, coffee)
	Carbonated beverages
	Cheese
	Acidic juices
	Tomatoes
	Vinegar
	Spicy foods—onions, garlic, etc.

the fact that in 2005, $3.5 billion was spent on over-the-counter (OTC) treatment for the common cold.[36] Initial treatment of chronic rhinosinusitis usually involves tailored appropriate medical therapy that may include protracted antimicrobial therapy (4 or more weeks), as well as multiple medications aimed at reducing inflammation. These may include topical intranasal steroids or systemic steroids, antihistamines, and leukotriene modifiers. Antifungal medications, both topical and systemic, may also be useful in selected patients with fungal involvement. Patients who experience head pain with their rhinosinusitis may self-medicate with over-the-counter nonsteroidal anti-inflammatory agents (NSAIDs). Patients who fail optimal medical treatment may be candidates for functional endoscopic sinus surgery (FESS) to improve sinus ventilation and drainage. Endoscopic sinus surgery has been found to be very effective in alleviating symptoms.[37,38]

Clinicians treating upper respiratory problems are reminded that older antihistamines such as diphenhydramine (Benadryl®) that have stronger anticholinergic effects in addition to their antihistamine function and can reduce the secretion and motility of the gastrointestinal system. This coupled with decongestants like pseudoephedrine (Sudafed®) may also worsen reflux in some individuals. The principle mechanism of action pseudoephedrine as a decongestant for the nose is the release of endogenous norepinephrine from storage vesicles in presynaptic neurons leading to vasoconstriction. Its effect on LES tone is less clearly stated in the literature but will have both α-adrenergic and β-adrenergic effects. Some patients notice reflux while on pseudoephedrine. Other medications that are α-blockers and β-agonists relax the LES and can exacerbate the tendency to gastric reflux. Beta-adrenergic agonists are a class of drugs commonly used as bronchodilators to treat asthma and other pulmonary disease states. Alpha-blockers are commonly used to treat: benign prostatic hyperplasia (BPH), high blood pressure (hypertension), and symptoms of non inflammatory chronic pelvic pain syndrome.[39,40] Xanthines, including caffeine and theophyline (which is still used to treat asthma) both relax smooth muscle of the lungs.[41] They also increase production of gastric acid and pepsin and are associated with worsening GER. Systemic steroids are commonly used to reduce inflammation of sinusitis or asthma and in higher doses or in combination with NSAIDs, hypoalbuminemia, or cirrhosis there is an association with peptic ulceration.[42]

One medication that raises concern for the authors of this chapter is the widespread use of guaifenesin. It is a commonly used, generally safe, over-the-counter expectorant and mucus thinner. It is used as a single agent or in combination with many other "cold preparations" and to treat postnasal drip. The mechanism of action is through irritation of gastric vagal receptors, and recruitment of efferent parasympathetic reflexes that cause glandular exocytosis of a less viscous mucus mixture. This may provoke cough.[43] Thus, treating upper respiratory disorders with guaifenesin theoretically could result in exacerbations of baseline reflux by increasing gastric acid secretion and promoting cough with attendant elevations in intra-abdominal pressure. This therefore can exacerbate the tendency to reflux. Studies are warranted to determine the significance of this condition as it relates to reflux.

EVIDENCE SUPPORTING EER TO SINUS AND MIDDLE EAR INFLAMMATION

Although much of the initial literature investigating EER has concentrated on its association with lower airway and laryngeal manifestations, more attention has recently been directed to the upper airways and sinuses. This may be because laryngeal irritation associated with reflux often appears to be more specific in its presentation than its association with other evidence of EER. For example, irritation of the larynx may actually be severe enough to cause intermittent laryngospasm, resulting in sustained vocal fold adduction, and momentary physiologic airway obstruction. This is typically followed by a slow return to normal breathing.[44] Although GER may present with classic "heartburn," more common laryngeal symptoms of LPR include mild hoarseness, frequent throat clearing, chronic cough, globus pharyngeus, and excessive mucus production.[45] Belafsky et al[46] developed the self-administered Reflux Symptom Index (RSI) to assist in quantifying symptom severity, in addition to evaluating treatment response. Koufman noted that throat clearing was a complaint of 87% of patients with LPR, compared to 3% of GER patients. Although only 20% of LPR patients complained of classic heartburn, as compared to 83% of those with GER.[2] There are multiple clinical findings suggestive of LPR, of which laryngeal erythema and edema on laryngoscopic examination may be the most commonly noted.[47–49] Challenges exist with regard to accepting varied physical finding as the method to diagnosis of LPR since the specificity of laryngeal findings of LPR has been questioned. In one important study 87% of healthy volunteers have been noted to have clinical findings previously suggestive of LPR,[50] thereby making it difficult to assert diagnosis of disease based on upper airway findings alone in the adult.

Several adult studies have demonstrated a relationship between gastric reflux and chronic rhinosinusitis. In 1997, Chambers[51] noted gastroesophageal reflux to be a predictor of poor symptomatic outcome after functional endoscopic sinus surgery. DiBaise has performed multiple studies on this topic as well. He first demonstrated a high prevalence of gastroesophageal reflux in patients with CRS; they found that 78% of patients had gastroesophageal reflux based on esophageal pH monitoring, and that 67% of patients experienced symptomatic improvement after treatment for GER.[52] More recently, in a small prospective study, DiBaise demonstrated a high prevalence (81.8%) of gastroesophageal reflux in patients with CRS unresponsive to conventional medical and surgical therapy.[53] Similarly, Ulualp et al[54] demonstrated a significantly higher prevalence of pharyngeal acid reflux in patients with CRS unresponsive to therapy as compared to controls. Further evidence of this association was noted by DelGaudio[55] when he documented the presence of nasopharyngeal reflux (NPR) in patients with CRS. He found that patients with persistent refractory CRS after endoscopic sinus surgery have more reflux at the nasopharynx, upper esophageal sphincter, and distal esophagus than controls. The greatest difference was noted with the nasopharyngeal reflux, especially when a pH less than 5 was used. This is the first study to demonstrate a significant difference in nasopharyngeal reflux of gastric acid in patients with refractory CRS as compared to controls.[55]

Several pediatric studies have suggested an association between reflux and chronic rhinosinusitis. Contencin and Narcy[56] studied children with recurrent or chronic rhinitis, and rhinopharyngitis, as compared to controls. They measured nasopharyngeal reflux (NPR) using 24-hour pH nasopharyngeal probes, and measured NPR episodes as a pH drop below 6. They concluded that the study group had significantly more NPR episodes and percentage of study time below pH 6.0 than controls. A limitation of this study is that an esophageal sensor was not used in combination with the nasopharyngeal sensor.[56] This, of course, would have allowed confirmation of true reflux episodes by noting a preceding drop of the esophageal probe prior to a drop at the nasopharyngeal probe. In addition, a pH of 6 was used a positive value rather than 4 or 5.[56] Barbero[57] has described several cases in which patients with intractable rhinosinusitis and otitis media have improved with reflux therapy. Beste et al[58] also noted that reflux may be a complicating factor in patients undergoing repair of bilateral choanal atresia. They documented post-operative reflux in all four of the patients included in the study, and noted that these patients required multiple dilations and prolonged stenting of their choanal atresia. In a retrospective study, Bothwell et al[59] noted that 89% of pediatric patients (25 of 28) with chronic rhinosinusitis were able to avoid functional endoscopic sinus surgery after subsequent treatment of their reflux disease. A prospective pediatric study by Phipps et al[60] studied 30 children with chronic rhinosinusitis refractory to medical treatment. All participants underwent 24-hour dual pH studies with sensors in both the esophagus and nasopharynx. Positive reflux episodes were noted with a pH drop below 4. Results of this study showed that 63% of patients demonstrated esophageal reflux, whereas 32% had nasopharyngeal reflux. Moreover, 79% of patients showed improvement of CRS symptoms after aggressive reflux treatment.[60]

Keles et al[61] reported a prospective study to investigate the association between pharyngeal reflux and adenoid hyperplasia by using 24-hr esophageal pH monitoring with a dual probe in children. They evaluated 30 children with adenoid hyperplasia, and a control group of 12 healthy children.[61] All children underwent 24-hr esophageal pH monitoring with a dual probe (distal and proximal esophageal pH monitoring). In the children with adenoidal hypertrophy the frequency of pharyngeal reflux was 46.7% and the gastroesophageal reflux (GER) was 64.5%, whereas, in the control group, they were 8.3% and 25%, respectively. There was a significant difference between study and control groups for frequencies of pharyngeal reflux and GER.[61] Another study by Mandell and Yellon[62] sought to determine the incidence of synchronous airway lesions in 35 children under 18 months of age undergoing adenoidectomy. They found synchronous airway lesions in 19 (59%) of 32 patients who underwent airway endoscopy. Interestingly they found histologic evidence of gastroesophageal reflux disease was found in 10 patients (31%), and eosinophilic esophagitis was found in 4 patients (13%). Overall prevalence of any synchronous finding (airway and/or esophagus) was 27 (77%) of 35.[62]

Multiple pediatric studies have also described an association between reflux and chronic otitis media. Otitis media (OM) is one of the most common medical conditions in the pediatric population, and can lead to hearing loss, delayed speech development, and permanent middle ear damage.[63] Otitis media has actually been shown to have the highest reported incidence among all medical conditions in children less than 5 years of age.[64] Multiple etiologies have been proposed as the cause of OM, including GER. Two studies by Tasker et al[10,65] suggest a correlation between reflux and OM. They found 83% and 91% of patients undergoing typanostomy for otitis media with effusion (OME) or glue ear had detectable pepsin/pepsinogen in the middle ear fluid in concentrations 1000-fold greater than that found in normal serum. In addition, no evidence of pepsin production was noted in 3 middle ear biopsy specimens.[10] A study by Lieu et al[66] confirmed this association between OM and reflux. They detected pepsin/pepsinogen in 77% of middle ear aspirates from children undergoing typanostomy tube placement for recurrent or chronic otitis media; however, questionnaire data provided by the parents did not show a prevalence of GER symptoms in the same pediatric patients. More recently, two other studies have demonstrated a lower incidence of pepsin in children with otitis media (14.4% and 20%, respectively).[67,68] The assay methods used to determine the presence of pepsin in these two studies were different from the assays used in the prior studies where the incidence was found to be higher. Interestingly, pepsin was more likely to be detected in patients who were infants and in those who had a purulent effusion in one study with a control group.

DIAGNOSTIC TESTS

None of the standard techniques for pH monitoring to assert severity of GERD have been found universally applicable to detection of NPR. Nonetheless, 24-hr catheter-based esophageal pH monitoring is widely available and the traditional method of detection for GERD.[69] Unfortunately, the nasally passed pH catheter is uncomfortable and conspicuous, leading some patients to significantly restrict their daily activities or not complete the study. In some instances, patients may remain at home and consume a very limited diet while the catheter is in place.[69] Position of the sensing electrode can be erroneous, and either proximal or distal migration may alter the diagnosis. In addition, esophageal acid exposure may fluctuate from day to day.[69] The Bravo wireless pH-monitoring system was developed to circumvent the requirement for an uncomfortable and conspicuous transnasal catheter.[69] The Bravo wireless pH-monitoring system uses a radiotelemetry pH-sensing capsule attached to the mucosa of the distal esophagus.[69] A newer technology referred to as combined multichannel intraluminal impedance and pH, overcomes the major limitation inherent to all pH-monitoring systems, which is that they focus on acid exposure as the only measure of reflux.[69] By measuring intraluminal impedence the direction of refluxate can be determined and the clinician can distinguish swallow-related reflux events thereby improving accuracy. It can also determine minor changes in acidity or alkalinity of reflux events.[55] Currently, only combined multichannel intraluminal impedance-pH monitoring can discriminate nonacid reflux and direction of bolus transit. Unfortunately this remains catheter-based with inherent limitations of patient's tolerability and monitoring time (<24 hours).[69]

The main outcome measure of a pH-monitoring study is the extent of esophageal acid exposure calculated as a percentage of the day with esophageal pH less than 4.[69] Pepsin maintains some enzymatic activity up to a pH of 7[10-12] and pH of 6.9[3,4] is thought to be the lower limit of normal for mucous of the nasopharynx. Therefore, as mentioned previously, some researchers have shifted the threshold for diagnosis of acid NPR to higher than pH for detection purposes. Diagnostic testing for EER, especially involving the paranasal sinuses, is somewhat controversial, and not well defined. However, triple-pH probe testing in the lower esophagus, above the cricopharyngeus, and most importantly, in the nasopharynx, may provide the most accurate information regarding EER contributing to CRS. Prior to such an extensive and expensive evaluation however, an empiric therapeutic trial of PPI therapy for up to 6 months has been advised. Some contend if symptoms are severe or refractory after a 3-month trial additional evaluation of the esophagus and stomach is indicated. Recently an assay to detect nasal pepsin was trialed in a controlled, prospective study in 33 CRS patients and 20 controls without rhinosinusitis. The fluorometric pepsin assay correlated to the results of 24-hour dual-probe monitoring for LPR diagnosis with a 100% sensitivity and 92.5% specificity. Unfortunately, 55% of normal control subjects had reflux. Ozmen et al[70] suggest that perhaps this fluorometric technology could be used for LPR screening.

TREATMENT

Aggressive treatment of reflux should be considered in patients with recalcitrant CRS secondary to EER as there is only minimal mucosal protection in the proximal upper aerodigestive tract. Treatment is similar to that of LPR, and should begin with conservative measures. Lifestyle changes and behavioral modifications may include smoking cessation, low-fat diet, weight loss, more frequent intake of smaller meals, avoiding lying supine within 3 hours of eating, and avoiding bedtime snacks. Patients should also avoid foods such as chocolate, mint, cheese, acidic juices, caffeinated beverages, soda, and alcohol which may aggravate reflux. In addition, patients should avoid medications, such as nonsteroidal anti-inflammatory medications (NSAIDS) and bisphosphonates, which may also worsen reflux. Many common over-the-counter medications (OTC) and vitamin supplements may also worsen reflux in sensitive individuals (see Tables 9–3 and 9–4).

Medical treatment for reflux usually begins with antacids and histamine-2 receptor antagonists that have demonstrated response rates of 50%.[71,72] Prokinetic agents, such as metoclopramide, may also be used. These medications may increase esophageal motility, increase lower esophageal sphincter tone, and promote gastric emptying.[44] The mainstay of treatment, however, consists of proton-pump inhibitor (PPI) therapy. These medications act directly on the H+-K+ ATPase, the key enzyme in acid production in the parietal cells. PPIs are best taken 30 to 60 minutes prior to meals to allow for maximal concentration of medication prior to the activation of the food intake-stimulated proton pumps.[45] Optimal dosage of PPIs is somewhat controversial. In the series by DeBaise mentioned earlier, many patients experienced modest symptom improvement with twice-daily omeprazole treatment for 3 months.[53] Improvement seemed to peak at about 8 weeks, however, complete resolution of symptoms occurred infrequently.[53] Pincus et al[73] also noted symptomatic improvement in patients with recalcitrant CRS after antireflux therapy with proton-pump inhibitors. Park et al[74] demonstrated that bid therapy was superior to daily dosing. They noted a 50% response rate after 2 months of BID treatment, and a 70% overall response rate after 4 months. Others recommend a 6-month trial of treatment of bid therapy.[75] Recent evidence has demonstrated that long-term PPI therapy, particularly at high doses, may lead to an increased risk of hip fracture.[76] This is hypothesized to be secondary to decreased calcium absorption secondary to acid suppression. Thus, it is important to inform patients of this risk, and consider placing them on calcium and vitamin D supplementation while on long-term PPI therapy. Although the data are somewhat unclear, it may also be reasonable to add a histamine-2-receptor antagonist to BID PPI therapy at bedtime to control nocturnal acid breakthrough.[45,77] If patients continue to be unresponsive to aggressive medical treatment, then further evaluation of the reflux etiology, such as gastroesoduodenal reflux, should be considered. This may include: esophagogastroduodenoscopy (EGD), Bravo study, impedence-pH testing, manometry or motility studies. Antireflux surgery may also be a treatment option; however, the best results are noted in patients who respond favorably to medical therapy.[78]

SUMMARY

In summary, disorders such as CRS or otitis media and their medical therapies are associated with EER. The physiologic mechanisms by which this is known to be possible are described in this chapter. The very treatments used for common airway problems can induce reflux in predisposed individuals. Given the emerging evidence, refractory rhinosinusitis or refractory middle ear disease must herald suspicion of a relationship with silent reflux in the proper clinical setting. Documenting the existence of these associations can be vexing for a patient and clinician. Therefore, empiric therapy based on careful history and physical examination including upper airway endoscopy is often warranted. Failure or refractoriness of empiric trial with proton pump inhibition warrants further evaluation of the esophagus and stomach. This may include pH probe study, impedance measurements, evaluations of motility, and/or EGD. Whether or not preventive measures or medical therapy aimed at EER should be initiated as part of standard treatment for CRS and otitis media requires additional investigation. Should it be found helpful to initiate such treatments before or after sinus surgery or myringotomy, the positive impact on patient wellness and health care spending could be very significant. Additional research is needed to improve our ability to comfortably and reliably detect pH in the sinonasal passages as well as to detect pepsin activity on the surfaces of respiratory epithelium. Research that discerns the influence of medications used to treat CRS, asthma, and allergy could be helpful as well in understanding the role of reflux. Treatments that assist with restoring mucociliary protective mechanisms are likely to be very beneficial to restoring normal sinus and middle ear function.

REFERENCES

1. Pandolfino JE, Richter JE, Ours T, et al. Ambulatory esophageal pH monitoring using a wireless system. *Am J Gastroenterol.* 2003;98:740-749.
2. Koufman JA. The otolaryngologic manifestations of gastroesophageal reflux disease (GERD): a clinical investigation of 225 patients using ambulatory 24-hour pH monitoring and an experimental investigation of the role of acid and pepsin in the development of laryngeal injury. *Laryngoscope.* 1991;101(4 pt 2, suppl 53):1-78.
3. Luk CK, Dulfano MJ. Effect of pH, viscosity and ionic strength changes on ciliary beat frequency of human bronchial explants. *Clin Sci.* 1983;64:449-451.
4. Karnad DR, Mhaisekar DG, Moralwar KV. Respiratory mucus pH in tracheostomized intensive care unit patients: effects of colonization and pneumonia. *Crit Care Med.* 1990;18:699-701.
5. Mirza N, Lanza DC. The nasal airway and obstructed breathing during sleep. *Otolaryngol Clin North Am.* 1999;32(2):243-262.
6. Senior BA, Khan M, Schwimmer C, Rosenthal L, Benninger M. Gastroesophageal reflux and obstructive sleep apnea. *Laryngoscope.* 2001;111(12):2144-2146.

7. Wise SK, Wise JC, DelGaudio JM. Gastroesophageal reflux and laryngopharyngeal reflux in patients with sleep-disordered breathing. *Otolaryngol Head Neck Surg.* 2006;135(2):253-257.
8. Goyal RK. In: Brauawald E, Hauser SL, Fauci AS, Longo DL, Kasper DL, Jameson JL, eds. *Disease of the Esophagus in Harrison's Principles of Internal Medicine.* Vol 2. 15th ed. New York, NY: McGraw-Hill; 2001:1642-1649.
9. Wise SK, Wise JC, DelGaudio JM. Association of nasopharyngeal and laryngopharyngeal reflux with postnasal drip symptomatology in patients with and without rhinosinusitis. *Am J Rhinol.* 2006;20(3): 283-289.
10. Tasker A, Dettmar PW, Panetti M, Koufman JA, P Birchall J, Pearson JP. Is gastric reflux a cause of otitis media with effusion in children? *Laryngoscope.* 2002; 112(11):1930-1934.
11. Piper DW, Fenton BH. pH stability and activity curves of pepsin with special reference to their clinical importance. *Gut.* 1965;6(5):506-508.
12. Panetti M, Pearson JP, Dettmar PW, et al. Active pepsin in airway secretions: possible evidence for new supraesophaeal pH criteria. *Gastroenterology.* 2001;120: A118-A119.
13. Dobhan R, Castell DO. Normal and abnormal proximal esophageal acid exposure: results of ambulatory dual-probe pH monitoring. *Am J Gastroenterol.* 1993;88(1):25-29.
14. Meltzer EO, Hamilos DL, Hadley JA, Lanza DC, et al. Rhinosinusitis: developing guidance for clinical trials. *J Allergy Clin Immunol.* 2006;118(5 suppl):S17-S61.
15. Johnston N, Dettmar PW, Lively MO, et al. Effect of pepsin on laryngeal stress protein (Sep 70, Sep 53, and Hsp 70) response: role in laryngopharyngeal reflux disease. *Ann Otol Rhinol Laryngol.* 2006;115:47-58.
16. Johnston N, Knight J, Dettmar PW, Lively MO, Koufman J. Pepsin and carbonic anhydrase isoenzyme II as diagnostic marker for laryngopharyngreal reflux disease. *Laryngoscope.* 2004;114:2129-2134.
17. Loehrl TA, Smith TL. Chronic sinusitis and gastroesophageal reflux: are they related? *Curr Opin Otolaryngol Head Neck Surg.* 2004;12(1):18-20.
18. Lodi U, Harding SM, Coghlan HC, Guzzo MR, Walker LH. Autonomic regulation in asthmatics with gastroesophageal reflux. *Chest.* 1997;111(1):65-70.
19. Harding SM, Schan CA, Guzzo MR, Alexander RW, Bradley LA, Richter JE. Gastroesophageal reflux-induced bronchoconstriction. Is microaspiration a factor? *Chest.* 1995;108(5):1220-1227.
20. Loehrl TA, Smith TL, Darling RJ, et al. Autonomic dysfunction, vasomotor rhinitis, and extraesophageal manifestations of gastroesophageal reflux. *Otolaryngol Head Neck Surg.* 2002;126(4):382-387.
21. Alper J. Ulcers as an infectious disease. *Science.* 1993;260(5105):159-160.
22. Ozdek A, Cirak MY, Samim E, Bayiz U, Safak MA, Turet S. A possible role of Helicobacter pylori in chronic rhinosinusitis: a preliminary report. *Laryngoscope.* 2003;113(4):679-682.
23. Dinis PB, Subtil J. Helicobacter pylori and laryngopharyngeal reflux in chronic rhinosinusitis. *Otolaryngol Head Neck Surg.* 2006;134(1):67-72.
24. Kim HY, Dhong HJ, Chung SK, Chung KW, Chung YJ, Jang KT. Intranasal Helicobacter pylori colonization does not correlate with the severity of chronic rhinosinusitis. *Otolaryngol Head Neck Surg.* 2007;136(3):390-395.
25. Bluestone CD. Studies in otitis media: Children's Hospital of Pittsburgh—University of Pittsburgh Progress Report—2004. *Laryngoscope.* 2004;114(suppl 105):1-26.
26. Wittenborg MH, Neuhauser EB. Simple roentenographic demonstration of eustachian tubes and abnormalities. *AJR Radium Ther Nucl Med.* 1963;89: 1194-1200.
27. Moody SA, Alper CM, Doyle WJ. Daily tympanometry in children during the

cold season: association of otitis media with upper respiratory tract infections. *Int J Pediatr Otorhinolaryngol.* 1998; 45:143-150.

28. Lanza DC, Kennedy DW. Adult rhinosinusitis defined. *Otolaryngol Head Neck Surg.* 1997;117(3 pt 2):S1-S7.
29. Lund VJ, Kennedy DW. Quantification for staging sinusitis. The Staging and Therapy Group. *Ann Otol Rhinol Laryngol Suppl.* 1995;167:17-21.
30. Benninger MS, Ferguson BJ, Hadley JA, et al. Adult chronic rhinosinusitis: definitions, diagnosis, epidemiology, and pathophysiology. *Otolaryngol Head Neck Surg.* 2003;129(3 suppl):S1-S32.
31. Guarderas JC. Rhinitis and sinusitis: office management. *Mayo Clin Proc.* 1996; 71(9):882-888.
32. Ray NF, Baraniuk JN, Thamer M, et al. Healthcare expenditures for sinusitis in 1996: contributions of asthma, rhinitis, and other airway disorders. *J Allergy Clin Immunol.* 1999;103(3 pt 1):408-414.
33. Lucas JW, Schiller JS, Benson V. Summary health statistics for U.S. adults: National Health Interview Survey, 2001. *Vital Health Stat 10.* 2004(218):1-134.
34. Benninger MS, Sedory Holzer SE, Lau J. Diagnosis and treatment of uncomplicated acute bacterial rhinosinusitis: summary of the Agency for Health Care Policy and Research evidence-based report. *Otolaryngol Head Neck Surg.* 2000;122(1): 1-7.
35. Pynnonen MA, Terrell JE. Conditions that masquerade as chronic rhinosinusitis: a medical record review. *Arch Otolaryngol Head Neck Surg.* 2006;132(7):748-751.
36. Teresa R, Melanie B, Leigh S. Over-the-counter cough and cold medication use in young children. *Pediatric Nursing.* 2008;34(2):174-180,184.
37. Levine HL. Functional endoscopic sinus surgery: evaluation, surgery, and follow-up of 250 patients. *Laryngoscope.* 1990; 100(1):79-84.
38. Senior BA, Kennedy DW, Tanabodee J, Kroger H, Hassab M, Lanza D. Long-term results of functional endoscopic sinus surgery. *Laryngoscope.* 1998;108(2):151-157.
39. Adrenergic drugs and acid reflux. Retrieved May 1, 2008 from: http://acid-reflux-relief.blogspot.com/2007/10/adrenergic-drugs-and-acid-reflux.html
40. Tatro DS, ed. Drug interaction facts. St. Louis, MO: *Facts and Comparisons*, 1987: 298-300b. http://www.drugs.com/mmx/antihistamines-decongestants-and-anticholinergics.html
41. Rall T, Haynes RC, Murad F. Central nervous system stimulants and adrenocorticotropic hormone. In: *Goodman and Gilman's Pharmacological Basis of Therapeutics.* 6th ed. Toronto, Canada: Macmillan Publishing Co Inc.; 1980:595-596,1483.
42. Williams GH, Dluhy RG. Disorders of the adrenal cortex. In: Brauawald E, Hauser SL, Fauci AS, Longo DL, Kasper DL, Jameson JL, eds. *Harrison's Principles of Internal Medicine.* Vol 2. 15th ed. New York, NY: McGraw-Hill; 2001:2104.
43. Showing drug card for Guaifenesin (DB00874). Drug Bank. Retrieved May 1, 2008 from: http://www.drugbank.ca/cgi-bin/getCard.cgi?CARD=DB00874.txt
44. Divi V, Benninger MS. Diagnosis and management of laryngopharyngeal reflux disease. *Curr Opin Otolaryngol Head Neck Surg.* 2006;14(3):124-127.
45. Bove MJ, Rosen C. Diagnosis and management of laryngopharyngeal reflux disease. *Curr Opin Otolaryngol Head Neck Surg.* 2006;14(3):116-123.
46. Belafsky PC, Postma GN, Koufman JA. Validity and reliability of the reflux symptom index (RSI). *J Voice.* 2002;16(2): 274-277.
47. Qadeer MA, Swoger J, Milstein C, et al. Correlation between symptoms and laryngeal signs in laryngopharyngeal reflux. *Laryngoscope.* 2005;115(11):1947-1952.
48. Belafsky PC, Postma GN, Koufman JA. The validity and reliability of the reflux finding score (RFS). *Laryngoscope.* 2001; 111(8):1313-1317.

49. Hickson C, Simpson CB, Falcon R. Laryngeal pseudosulcus as a predictor of laryngopharyngeal reflux. *Laryngoscope.* 2001;111(10):1742-1745.
50. Hicks DM, Ours TM, Abelson TI, Vaezi MF, Richter JE. The prevalence of hypopharynx findings associated with gastroesophageal reflux in normal volunteers. *J Voice.* 2002;16(4):564-579.
51. Chambers DW, Davis WE, Cook PR, Nishioka GJ, Rudman DT. Long-term outcome analysis of functional endoscopic sinus surgery: correlation of symptoms with endoscopic examination findings and potential prognostic variables. *Laryngoscope.* 1997;107(4):504-510.
52. DiBaise JK, Huerter JV, Quigley EM. Sinusitis and gastroesophageal reflux disease. *Ann Intern Med.* 1998;129(12):1078.
53. DiBaise JK, Olusola BF, Huerter JV, Quigley EM. Role of GERD in chronic resistant sinusitis: a prospective, open label, pilot trial. *Am J Gastroenterol.* 2002;97(4):843-850.
54. Ulualp SO, Toohill RJ, Hoffmann R, Shaker R. Possible relationship of gastroesophagopharyngeal acid reflux with pathogenesis of chronic sinusitis. *Am J Rhinol.* 1999;13(3):197-202.
55. DelGaudio JM. Direct nasopharyngeal reflux of gastric acid is a contributing factor in refractory chronic rhinosinusitis. *Laryngoscope.* 2005;115(6):946-957.
56. Contencin P, Narcy P. Nasopharyngeal pH monitoring in infants and children with chronic rhinopharyngitis. *Int J Pediatr Otorhinolaryngol.* 1991;22(3):249-256.
57. Barbero GJ. Gastroesophageal reflux and upper airway disease. *Otolaryngol Clin North Am.* 1996;29(1):27-38.
58. Beste DJ, Conley SF, Brown CW. Gastroesophageal reflux complicating choanal atresia repair. *Int J Pediatr Otorhinolaryngol.* 1994;29(1):51-58.
59. Bothwell MR, Parsons DS, Talbot A, Barbero GJ, Wilder B. Outcome of reflux therapy on pediatric chronic sinusitis. *Otolaryngol Head Neck Surg.* 1999;121(3):255-262.
60. Phipps CD, Wood WE, Gibson WS, Cochran WJ. Gastroesophageal reflux contributing to chronic sinus disease in children: a prospective analysis. *Arch Otolaryngol Head Neck Surg.* 2000;126(7):831-836.
61. Keles B, Ozturk K, Arbag H, Gunel E, Ozer B. Frequency of pharyngeal reflux in children with adenoid hyperplasia. *Int J Pediatr Otorhinolaryngol.* 2005;69(8):1103-1107 [Epub Apr 18. 2005].
62. Mandell DL, Yellon RF. Synchronous airway lesions and esophagitis in young patients undergoing adenoidectomy. *Arch Otolaryngol Head Neck Surg.* 2007;133(4):375-378.
63. Bastos I, Janzon L, Lundgren K, Reimer A. Otitis media and hearing loss in children attending an ENT clinic in Luanda, Angola. *Int J Pediatr Otorhinolaryngol.* 1990;20(2):137-148.
64. Benson V, Marano MA. Current estimates from the National Health Interview Survey, 1995. *Vital Health Stat 10.* 1998;199:1-428.
65. Tasker A, Dettmar PW, Panetti M, Koufman JA, Birchall JP, Pearson JP. Reflux of gastric juice and glue ear in children. *Lancet.* 2002;359(9305):493.
66. Lieu JE, Muthappan PG, Uppaluri R. Association of reflux with otitis media in children. *Otolaryngol Head Neck Surg.* 2005;133(3):357-361.
67. He Z, O'Reilly RC, Bolling L, et al. Detection of gastric pepsin in middle ear fluid of children with otitis media. *Otolaryngol Head Neck Surg.* 2007;137(1):59-64.
68. O'Reilly RC, He Z, Bloedon E, et al. The role of extraesophageal reflux in otitis media in infants and children. *Laryngoscope.* 2008;118(7 pt2, suppl 116):1-9.
69. Kwiatek MA, Pandolfino JE. Prolonged reflux monitoring: capabilities of bravo pH and impedance-pH systems. *Current GERD Reports.* 2007;1(3):165-170.

70. Ozmen S, Yücel OT, Sinici I, et al. Nasal pepsin assay and pH monitoring in chronic rhinosinusitis. *Laryngoscope.* 2008;118(5):890-894.
71. Smith JT, Gavey C, Nwokolo CU, Pounder RE. Tolerance during 8 days of high-dose H2-blockade: placebo-controlled studies of 24-hour acidity and gastrin. *Aliment Pharmacol Ther.* 1990;4(suppl 1):47-63.
72. Wilder-Smith CH, Ernst T, Gennoni M, Zeyen B, Halter F, Merki HS. Tolerance to oral H2-receptor antagonists. *Dig Dis Sci.* 1990;35(8):976-983.
73. Pincus RL, Kim HH, Silvers S, Gold S. A study of the link between gastric reflux and chronic sinusitis in adults. *Ear Nose Throat J.* 2006;85(3):174-178.
74. Park W, Hicks DM, Khandwala F, et al. Laryngopharyngeal reflux: prospective cohort study evaluating optimal dose of proton-pump inhibitor therapy and pretherapy predictors of response. *Laryngoscope.* 2005;115(7):1230-1238.
75. Postma GN, Johnson LF, Koufman JA. Treatment of laryngopharyngeal reflux. *Ear Nose Throat J.* 2002;81(9 suppl 2): 24-26.
76. Yang YX, Lewis JD, Epstein S, Metz DC. Long-term proton pump inhibitor therapy and risk of hip fracture. *JAMA.* 2006;296(24):2947-2953.
77. Peghini PL, Katz PO, Castell DO. Ranitidine controls nocturnal gastric acid breakthrough on omeprazole: a controlled study in normal subjects. *Gastroenterology.* 1998;115(6):1335-1339.
78. So JB, Zeitels SM, Rattner DW. Outcomes of atypical symptoms attributed to gastroesophageal reflux treated by laparoscopic fundoplication. *Surgery.* 1998;124(1): 28-32.

when a fundoplication for GERD was performed, postoperative manometry revealed that esophageal peristalsis was restored to normal in 35.7% and improved in 50% following the operation. This improvement in motility provides additional basis for the added benefit of surgical therapy in the management of extraesophageal reflux.

CHOICE OF OPERATION

Surgical options for the treatment of patients with extraesophageal reflux are no different than for those undergoing fundoplication for traditional GERD. Special consideration has to be made for patients with a large hiatal hernia, shortened esophagus, motility abnormality, or delayed gastric emptying. Careful preoperative evaluation and analysis of diagnostic studies will help the surgeon determine whether or not a complete or partial fundoplication would best suit the patient.

ENDOLUMINAL THERAPY

Liu[31] documented the effectiveness of endoscopic therapy for atypical GERD symptoms. They treated 39 patients with symptoms of hoarseness, cough, and wheezing, after failing medical antisecretory therapy. Most were treated with the EndoCinch and a few with the flexible Endoscopic Suturing Device. Both devices enable endoscopic suturing to achieve endoluminal gastroplication at the gastroesophageal junction. Hoarseness resolved in 12 of 19 at 6 months; at 12 months 5 more resolved, but 9 recurred. Cough resolved in 17 of 19 at 6 months; at 12 months 1 more resolved but 7 recurred. Wheezing resolved in 8 of 9 at 6 months; at 12 months 1 more resolved while 1 recurred. Twenty patients had repeat endoscopy an average of 10 months after the initial procedure. Eleven (55%) retained all the sutures initially placed.

COMPLICATIONS OF SURGERY

The risks and complications of antireflux surgery are theoretically the same whether treating primarily extraesophageal or classical GERD symptoms. There are currently no published studies specifically addressing this issue.

In general, complications are rare in patients undergoing fundoplication. Most of the complications are temporary and minor and are related to surgical intervention in general (urinary retention, wound infection, and ileus). Others are related specifically to the procedure or approach (splenic injury, perforation of the esophagus or stomach, and pneumothorax). Although pneumothorax may occur in about 1%, the rate of more serious solid organ or hollow viscus injuries is well below 0.5% in recent studies.

Bloating and increased flatus may occur in up to 30% of patients; however, fewer than 5% describe this symptom after 2 months. Postoperative dysphagia may occur in up to 20% of patients initially. A much smaller percentage of patients require dilation for this problem. Long-term dysphagia requiring repeated dilation or surgical revision is reported in less than 2%. The overall death rate with the operation is less than 0.2%.[32]

CONCLUSION

Both medical and surgical therapies have been used to treat extraesophageal manifestations of gastroesophageal reflux disease. Resolution or improvement of respiratory and laryngeal symptoms and decreased medication requirements have all been observed. The rate of atypical, extraesophageal symptom response to surgery is less than that seen for heartburn and other classic GERD symptoms, but is still quite high (75-80%). It is believed that the lower response rate might be due to the difficulty in preoperatively predicting the role of reflux in the etiology of these atypical symptoms. Diagnosis still remains elusive because both GERD and pulmonary disease are common in the human population and could coexist without a direct interaction. However, if GERD is a contributor to the pulmonary process, then antireflux surgery can improve or even resolve the pulmonary process in many patients. Since the causes and exacerbating factors of many pulmonary diseases are multifactorial, predictive variables can help identify subsets of patients who should respond dramatically to antireflux surgery.

REFERENCES

1. Novitsky YW, Zawacki JK, Irwin RS, French CT, Hussey VM, Callery MP. Chronic cough due to gastroesophageal reflux disease: efficacy of antireflux surgery. *Surg Endosc.* 2002;16(4):567-571.
2. Patti MG, Arcerito M, Tamburini A, et al. Effect of laparoscopic fundoplication on gastroesophageal reflux disease-induced respiratory symptoms. *J Gastrointest Surg.* 2000;4(2):143-149.
3. Greason KL, Miller DL, Deschamps C, et al. Effects of antireflux procedures on respiratory symptoms. *Ann Thorac Surg.* 2002;73(2):381-385.
4. Hunter JG, Trus TL, Branum GD, Waring JP, Wood WC. A physiologic approach to laparoscopic fundoplication for gastroesophageal reflux disease. *Ann Surg.* 1996; 223(6):673-685; discussion 685-677.
5. Brouwer R, Kiroff GK. Improvement of respiratory symptoms following laparoscopic Nissen fundoplication. *ANZ J Surg.* 2003;73(4):189-193.
6. DeMeester TR, Bonavina L, Iascone C, Courtney JV, Skinner DB. Chronic respiratory symptoms and occult gastroesophageal reflux. A prospective clinical study and results of surgical therapy. *Ann Surg.* 1990;211(3):337-345.
7. Oelschlager BK, Eubanks TR, Oleynikov D, Pope C, Pellegrini CA. Symptomatic and physiologic outcomes after operative treatment for extraesophageal reflux. *Surg Endosc.* 2002;16(7):1032-1036.
8. Wetscher GJ, Glaser K, Hinder RA, et al. Respiratory symptoms in patients with gastroesophageal reflux disease following medical therapy and following antireflux surgery. *Am J Surg.* 1997;174(6): 639-642; discussion 642-633.
9. Field SK, Gelfand GA, McFadden SD. The effects of antireflux surgery on asthmatics with gastroesophageal reflux. *Chest.* 1999;116(3):766-774.
10. Shaker R, Dodds WJ, Ren J, Hogan WJ, Arndorfer RC. Esophagoglottal closure reflex: a mechanism of airway protection. *Gastroenterology.* 1992;102(3):857-861.
11. Bowrey DJ, Peters JH, DeMeester TR. Gastroesophageal reflux disease in asthma: effects of medical and surgical antireflux therapy on asthma control. *Ann Surg.* 2000;231(2):161-172.
12. Spivak H, Smith CD, Phichith A, Galloway K, Waring JP, Hunter JG. Asthma and gastroesophageal reflux: fundoplication decreases need for systemic corticosteroids. *J Gastrointest Surg.* 1999;3(5): 477-482.

13. Ekstrom T, Johansson KE. Effects of antireflux surgery on chronic cough and asthma in patients with gastro-oesophageal reflux disease. *Respir Med.* 2000;94(12): 1166-1170.
14. Allen CJ, Anvari M. Gastro-oesophageal reflux related cough and its response to laparoscopic fundoplication. *Thorax.* 1998;53(11):963-968.
15. Wright RC, Rhodes KP. Improvement of laryngopharyngeal reflux symptoms after laparoscopic Hill repair. *Am J Surg.* 2003;185(5):455-461.
16. Salminen P, Sala E, Koskenvuo J, Karvonen J, Ovaska J. Reflux laryngitis: a feasible indication for laparoscopic antireflux surgery? *Surg Laparosc Endosc Percutan Tech.* 2007;17(2):73-78.
17. Swoger J, Ponsky J, Hicks DM, et al. Surgical fundoplication in laryngopharyngeal reflux unresponsive to aggressive acid suppression: a controlled study. *Clin Gastroenterol Hepatol.* 2006;4(4):433-441.
18. Perrin-Fayolle M, Gormand F, Braillon G, et al. Long-term results of surgical treatment for gastroesophageal reflux in asthmatic patients. *Chest.* 1989;96(1):40-45.
19. Kaufman JA, Houghland JE, Quiroga E, Cahill M, Pellegrini CA, Oelschlager BK. Long-term outcomes of laparoscopic antireflux surgery for gastroesophageal reflux disease (GERD)-related airway disorder. *Surg Endosc.* 2006;20(12):1824-1830.
20. Allen CJ, Anvari M. Does laparoscopic fundoplication provide long-term control of gastroesophageal reflux related cough? *Surg Endosc.* 2004;18(4):633-637.
21. Floch NR. Surgical therapy for atypical symptoms of GERD: patient selection and preoperative evaluation. *J Clin Gastroenterol.* 2000;30(3 suppl):S45-S47.
22. So JB, Zeitels SM, Rattner DW. Outcomes of atypical symptoms attributed to gastroesophageal reflux treated by laparoscopic fundoplication. *Surgery.* 1998; 124(1):28-32.
23. Johnson WE, Hagen JA, DeMeester TR, et al. Outcome of respiratory symptoms after antireflux surgery on patients with gastroesophageal reflux disease. *Arch Surg.* 1996;131(5):489-492.
24. Larrain A, Carrasco E, Galleguillos F, Sepulveda R, Pope CE, 2nd. Medical and surgical treatment of nonallergic asthma associated with gastroesophageal reflux. *Chest.* 1991;99(6):1330-1335.
25. Spechler SJ, Gordon DW, Cohen J, Williford WO, Krol W. The effects of antireflux therapy on pulmonary function in patients with severe gastroesophageal reflux disease. Department of Veterans Affairs Gastroesophageal Reflux Disease Study Group. *Am J Gastroenterol.* 1995; 90(6):915-918.
26. Sontag SJ, O'Connell S, Khandelwal S, et al. Asthmatics with gastroesophageal reflux: long term results of a randomized trial of medical and surgical antireflux therapies. *Am J Gastroenterol.* 2003; 98(5):987-999.
27. Patti MG, Debas HT, Pellegrini CA. Clinical and functional characterization of high gastroesophageal reflux. *Am J Surg.* 1993; 165(1):163-166; discussion 166-168.
28. Tibbling L. Wrong-way swallowing as a possible cause of bronchitis in patients with gastroesophageal reflux disease. *Acta Otolaryngol.* 1993;113(3):405-408.
29. Tutuian R, Mainie I, Agrawal A, Adams D, Castell DO. Nonacid reflux in patients with chronic cough on acid-suppressive therapy. *Chest.* 2006;130(2):386-391.
30. Knight RE, Wells JR, Parrish RS. Esophageal dysmotility as an important co-factor in extraesophageal manifestations of gastroesophageal reflux. *Laryngoscope.* 2000;110(9):1462-1466.
31. Liu JJ, Carr-Locke DL, Osterman MT, et al. Endoscopic treatment for atypical manifestations of gastroesophageal reflux disease. *Am J Gastroenterol.* 2006;101(3): 440-445.
32. Horgan S, Pellegrini CA. Surgical treatment of gastroesophageal reflux disease. *Surg Clin North Am.* 1997;77(5):1063-1082.

Index

A

ACEi (angiotensin-converting enzyme inhibitors), 110
Achalasia, 158
Alcohol, 23, 39, 42, 56, 69, 72, 139, 144
Alendronate, 139
Alpha adrenergic blockers, 139, 140
Amoxicillin, 138
Anosmia, 138
Antacids, 13, 56, 80, 100, 144, 201
Antibiotics, 138, 173
Anticholinergics, 139
Antifungal medications, 139
Antihistamines, 110, 138, 139, 173
Arrythmias, 2
Aspirin, 136, 139
Asthma
- diagnostic overview, 172–173
- as EERD manifestation of GERD, 2, 28, 172
  - biological plausibility, 7
  - and esophagitis, 26
  - and prevalence, 6–7
  - and reflux, 173
  - treatment, 7–8, 14
- and GERD
  - axonal reflexes, 96
  - biomarkers, 97
  - bronchoconstriction, 97
  - and bronchospasm, 95
  - epidemiology, 93–95
  - factors promoting, 95
  - GERD-induced lung responses, 95–98
  - microaspiration, esophageal contents, 96–97
  - nonacid reflux, 97–98
  - outcomes with GERD therapy, 98–100
  - overview, 93, 101–102
  - and pulmonary airflow, 97
  - treatment, 100–101
  - unanswered questions, 101
  - vagally mediated reflex, 96
- *Guidelines for the Diagnosis and Management of Asthma* (National Heart, Lung, and Blood Institute), 100
- and heartburn, 94

B

Baclofen, 59, 127–128
Barrett's esophagus, 20, 21, 55
Benadryl, 138, 139
Beta adrenergic agonists, 95, 138, 140
Bisphonates, 144
BPH (benign prostatic hyperplasia), 140
Bronchitis, 2, 3, 6, 26
Bronchodilators, 110, 140, 173
Bronchospasm, 95, 110
Burning sensation
- as EERD manifestation of GERD, 2
- and globus sensation, 80
- and LPR, 38
- in mouth, 12
- in throat, 38, 80
- in windpipe, 134

C

Caffeine, 42, 56, 57, 72, 138, 139, 140, 144
Calcium channel blockers, 139
Cancer
- as EERD manifestation of GERD, 2, 3
- and *Helicobacter pylori*, 22
- and LPR, 51, 53, 58

Carcinoma
  and *Helicobacter pylori*, 22
  and LPR, 38, 50–51, 67, 69, 71, 95
Causality, epidemiological
  analogy/explanatory evidence, 3–4
  Austin Bradford Hill criteria, 2–3
  and laboratory/clinical findings, 3, 13–14
  overview, 13–14
Cervical tension/LPR, 68, 73
Chest pain, noncardiac (NCCP)
  diagnostic overview, 175–176
  as EERD manifestation of GERD
    biological plausibility, 10–11, 14
    and prevalence, 10
    treatment, 11–12
Chocolate, 23, 42, 57, 139, 144
Chronic obstructive pulmonary disorder, 26
Cimetidine, 100
Clavulanate, 138
Clindamycin, 138
Cobblestoning, 29, 40, 53, 54
Corticosteroids, 95, 101, 173
Cough, chronic
  diagnostic overview, 173–175
  as EERD manifestation of GERD, 2, 28
    biological plausibility, 9
    and prevalence, 8-9, 26
    treatment, 8–10
  and GERD
    barium studies, 113
    bronchoscopy, 113–114
    diagnosis/treatment algorithm, 125–127
    diagnostic testing, 110–114
    endoscopy, 110–111
    epidemiology, 109
    future directions, 127–128
    impedance testing, 111–112
    laryngoscopy, 110–111
    manometry, 111–112
    nonacid reflux, 113
    overview, 107–108
    pathophysiology, 109–110
    pH monitoring, esophageal, 111–113
    treatment, 114–127
  and LPR, 37, 38, 39, 51, 52
CRS (chronic rhinosinusitis). *See* chronic *under* Rhinosinusitis

D

Dental enamel erosion, 2, 12, 13
Diagnosis
  asthma, 172–173
  biopsy, esophageal, 167
  cough, chronic, 173–175
  endoscopy, 167
  of ENT manifestations of GERD, 169
  GERD central contradiction, 1
  impedance, 167–168
  of laryngitis, 169–172
  laryngoscopy, 167
  LPR, 37–42, 50, 54–56, 72, 140–141
  nasopharyngeal reflux (NPR), 143–144
  pH monitoring, 166
  PPI trials, 168
  of pulmonary manifestations, 172
  sinonasal passages/middle ear and EERD, 143–144
Diazepam, 139
Diet, 23, 42, 56, 57, 72, 128, 139, 144
Diphenhydramine, 138, 139
Dysphagia
  as EERD manifestation of GERD, 2, 4
  from fundoplication, 158–160
  GERD
    and cricopharyngeal bar, 156
    and diffuse esophageal spasm, 158
    dysphagia as consequence of, 151–156, 158–161
    and eosinophilic esophagitis (EoE), 156–157
    and esophageal web, 156
    HGM (heterotopic gastric mucosa), 156
    nonobstructive, 153–155
    peptic strictures, 151–153
    and Schatzki's ring, 155–156
    and scleroderma, 157
    and upper esophagus, 156
    and Zenker's diverticulum, 156
  and LPR, 37, 38, 39, 68, 70
  nonobstructive, 153–155
  treatment

acid suppression medical therapy, 152–153, 154–155, 156, 158
dilation, 152–153
surgical, 155
Dysphonia. *See also* MTD (muscular tension dysphonia)
and globus, 86
and laryngospasm, 60
and LPR, 37, 38, 39, 51, 68
and upper respiratory infection, 85

E

EERD (extraesophageal reflux disease)
and acid suppression treatment, 1, 6, 7–8, 9–10, 11–12 (*See also* Treatment)
dental GERD manifestations, 12–13, 14
diagnostic algorithm, 176–178
dysphagia, 2, 4
ear symptoms, 134
and GERD manifestations, 2, 4–10, 12–13, 14
and GERD symptoms overview, 1–2, 178
and globus sensation, 80, 81
and laparoscopic fundoplication, 59
laryngeal symptoms, 134
nasal symptoms, 134
oral cavity symptoms, 134
otolaryngologic GERD manifestations, 4–6, 14
pathophysiology
bile acids and pancreatic enzymes, 26
and differential diagnosis, 28
esophagotracheobronchial cough reflex, 26, 27
gastric acid and pepsin, 26
and laryngeal injury from GERD, 28–31
and LPR, 28–31
and lung injury from GERD, 26–28
micro-/macroaspiration, esophageal reflux, 26–27
nonacid reflux (NAR), 27–28, 31
overview, 26
tracheobronchial reflex, 26–27
pharyngeal symptoms, 134
pulmonary GERD manifestations, 6–10, 14
pulmonary symptoms, 134
sinonasal passages/middle ear, 133–145 (*See also main heading* Sinonasal passages/middle ear)
diagnostic tests, 143–144
evidence supporting association, 140–143
otitis media (OM), 142–143
overview, 145
pharyngeal reflux, 142
treatment, 144–145
sinus symptoms, 134
tooth erosion GERD manifestations, 12–13
EGD (esophagogastroduodenoscopy), 79, 111, 145
Endoscopy. *See also* Transnasal endoscopy (TNE)
air-puff stimuli, 30
and cough, 110, 111, 119
diagnostic value, 86–87
as dysphagia etiology, 160–161
GERD and cough, 110–111
and GERD/noncardiac chest pain, 11
and LPR, 55, 58, 68–69
overview, 167
Epidemiology
asthma/GERD, 93–95
causality, epidemiological, 2–4 (*See also main heading* Causality, epidemiological)
and EERD manifestations of GERD, 13–14
prevalence
of asthma as EERD manifestation of GERD, 6–7
of chronic cough as EERD manifestation of GERD, 8–9, 26
of GERD, 1
of laryngitis as EERD manifestation of GERD, 4
of noncardiac chest pain as EERD manifestation of GERD, 10
of tooth erosion as EERD manifestation of GERD, 95
of wheezing as EERD manifestation of GERD, 26

Esomeprazole
for asthma, 8
for dysphagia, 153, 154
for GERD/asthma outcomes, 98
for GERD with cough, 115, 121
for laryngitis, 5, 171
for LPR, 42, 187, 188
for reflux laryngitis, 111
Esophageal spasm, diffuse, 158
Esophagitis
acid and pepsin, 20
endoscopic, 21
eosinophilic (EoE), 156-157
erosive, 110, 111
and esophageal clearance, 24-25
LES pressures low, 23
and pulmonary disease risk, 26
reflux, 151
Expectorants, 138

F

Fosamax, 139

G

Gastroenterology, laryngitis, 37-44. *See also main heading* Laryngitis; *main heading* LPR (laryngopharyngeal reflux)
GERD (gastroesophageal disease)
and ACEi (angiotensin-converting enzyme inhibitors), 110
and asthma
asthma medication use, 95
asthma outcomes/GERD therapy, 98-100
axonal reflexes, 96
biomarkers, 97
bronchoconstriction, 97
and bronchospasm, 95
factors promoting, 95
with GERD treatment, 100-101
microaspiration, esophageal contents, 96-97
nonacid reflux, 97-98
overview, 93, 101-102
and pulmonary airflow, 97
unanswered questions, 101
vagally mediated reflex, 96
and cough
barium studies, 113
bronchoscopy, 113-114
diagnosis/treatment algorithm, 125-127
diagnostic testing, 110-114
endoscopy, 110-111
epidemiology, 109
future directions, 127-128
impedance testing, 111-112
laryngoscopy, 110-111
manometry, 112
nonacid reflux, 113
overview, 107-108
pathophysiology, 109-110
treatment, 114-127
dysphagia, 151-161 (*See also* GERD *under* Dysphagia)
and EERD symptom overview, 1-2
epidemiology/asthma, 93-95
extraesophageal manisfestations, proposed, 2
fundoplication, laparoscopic Nissen, 113
and globus sensation, 79-80
and LPR, 50
versus LPR symptoms, 51
lung responses induced by, 95-98
management/asthma, 100-101
medical treatment, 185-186
and OSA, 51
over-the-counter (OTC) remedies, 56
over-the-counter remedies (*See also main heading* over-the-counter (OTC))
overview, 1
pathophysiology
acid and pepsin, 20
acid neutralization, esophageal clearance, 25
biliary and pancreatic secretions, 20-22
and EGF (epidermal growth factor), 25
epithelial defense/repair, esophageal clearance, 25
esophageal clearance, 24-25

gastric emptying, 22
gastroduodenal factors, 20–22
gastroesophageal junction factors, 22–24
Helicobacter pylori, 22
hiatal hernia, 24
hypotensive LES, 23
nonacid reflux (NAR), 22
overview, 19–20, 25–26
pepsin and acid, 20
pulmonary complaints, 26
TLESRs (transient LES relaxations), 22, 23
silent, 26, 108, 117
Globus sensation
and achalasia, 78
current practice review, 83–84
defined, 77–78
diagnostic testing, 86–87
and differential diagnosis, 84–85
and EERD, 2, 4, 26, 80, 81
and EGD (esophago-gastroduodenoscopy), 79
and esophageal dysmotility, 78–79
and esophageal stretch, 79
and GERD, 79–80
and hypochalasia, 78
and LPR, 37, 51, 52, 68
management, 87–88
and MBS (modified barium swallow), 87
and MTD (muscular tension dysphonia), 80–81
overview, 77, 88
and patient history, 84–85
and pH monitoring, 79–80
physical examination, 86
and proton-pump inhibitors (PPIs), 85
and psychological associations, 82–83
RSI score, 82
and stress triggers, 85
and transnasal endoscopy (TNE), 87
and trauma history, 84–85
and UES dysfunction, 78–79
and URI, 85
and weight loss, unintentional, 84
Granuloma
and LPR, 29, 40, 73
recurrent, 58
vocal fold, 53, 54, 69, 71
Guaifenesin, 138, 140
Guidelines for the Diagnosis and Management of Asthma (National Heart, Lung, and Blood Institute), 100

H

Halitosis, 2, 12, 134, 138
Heartburn
and asthma, 94
and EERD, 9
as episodic, 31
and esophageal reflux exposure, 20
and GERD, 1, 14, 25, 28, 51, 79
and globus sensation, 79
incidence, 19, 51
and laparoscopic fundoplication, 123
and LPR, 39, 42, 51, 67, 68
postprandial, 21
recurrent, 1, 19
Helicobacter pylori
GERD pathophysiology, 22
sinonasal passages, 136–137
Histamine-2 receptor antagonists (H2RA)
and chronic rhinosinusitus (CRS), 144
combination/PPIs, 43–44, 113
and cough, 113, 114
and erosive esophagitis, 111
and LPR, 43–44, 56, 58
for LPR, 186, 189
for sinonasal passages/middle ear involvement, 144
Hoarseness
as EERD manifestation of GERD, 2, 4, 26
and laryngoscopic examination need, 53
and LPR, 51, 52, 68
H2RA. *See* Histamine-2 receptor antagonists (H2RA)
Hyposmia, 138

I

Impedance, 111–112, 135, 145, 167–168
Iron supplements, 139

L

Lansoprazole
  as asthma treatment, 8, 97, 99
  for cough, 114, 115, 116, 117, 120, 121
  for GERD, 5, 11
    and asthma, 97
    with cough, 114, 115, 120, 121
  for laryngitis, 5, 171
  for LPR, 57, 187, 188
  for noncardiac chest pain, 11-12
  for noncardiac chest pain (NCCP), 176
Laryngeal edema, 29, 39
Laryngeal erythema and LPR, 39
Laryngeal hyperemia, 29
Laryngitis
  chronic posterior, 111
  diagnostic overview, 169-172
  as EERD manifestation of GERD
    biological plausibility, 4-5
    and prevalence, 4
    treatment, 5-6
  reflux, 37-44, 110, 111 (*See also* LPR (laryngopharyngeal reflux))
Laryngopharyngitis, 122
Laryngoscopy
  overview, 167
Laryngoscopy, GERD and cough, 110-111
Laryngospasm
  and LPR, 58, 67, 70, 71, 73-74
  overview, 70
  respiratory retraining, 73
  and vocal fold adduction, 140
Leukotriene modifiers, 139
Long-acting beta-agonists (LABAs), 98-99
LPR (laryngopharyngeal reflux). *See also* Dysphonia
  and biomarkers, molecular, 56
  and carcinoma, 50-51, 95
  and chronic rhinosinusitis (CRS), 138
  clinical manifestations, 39
  clinical presentation, 51-52
  diagnosis, 39-42, 54-56, 72
    challenges, 141
    controversy, 37-38
    and GERD, 39, 40
    laryngoscopy, 39-40, 41
    pH monitoring, 39-40, 40-42
    and pseudoreflux inclusion, 41
    and symptoms, 39, 41-42, 50, 140-141
  diagnosis controversy, 37-38
  dysphagia, 70
  and EERD, 28-31
  endoscopy, 55, 58, 63-69
  flurometric technology, 144
  and GERD, 39, 40, 50
  versus GERD symptoms, 51
  granuloma, vocal process, 69, 73
  head and neck disorders, 50-51
  laparoscopic Nissen-Rossetti fundoplication, 59
  laryngeal conditions, 68
  laryngospasm, 70, 73-74
  management, 42, 56-60 (*See also main heading* Treatment)
  and OSA, 51
  overview, 37-38, 44, 59-60, 67-68
  pathophysiology, 38-39, 49-50
  patient history, 51-52
  persistent symptoms with treatment, 39, 41-42, 50
  pH monitoring, 55-56
  physical findings, 52-54
  and PPIs, 41, 42-44
  and PPIs/H2RA, 43-44
  proton-pump inhibitors (PPIs), 37
  PVFM, 69-70, 73-74
  and RFS (Reflux Finding Score), 53-54, 58
  and RSI (Reflux Symptom Index), 39, 40, 52, 58, 140-141
  SLP role, 70-74 (*See main heading* SLP role, LPR)
  and symptoms, 39, 41-42, 50, 140-141
  and terminology, 37
  and transnasal endoscopy (TNE), 55, 58
  transnasal laryngoscopic findings, 52-54
  treatment, 37, 42, 72
    algorithm, 190
    drug therapy, 186-189
    overview, 186, 189
  and VAPP (Voice Activity and Participation Profile), 72
  and VHI (Voice Handicap Index), 72

videostrobolaryngoscopy, 68-69
voice conditions, 68

M

Manometry
dysphagia, nonobstructive, 153
esophageal dysmotility, 78
and esophageal spasm, diffuse, 158
esophagoglottal closure reflex, 30
and globus management, 87
hiatal hernia, 24
and impedance, 112
LPR, 55, 58
and Schatzki's ring, 155
and scleroderma, 157
sinonasal passages/middle ear, 145
MBS (modified barium swallow), globus sensation, 80, 87
Metoclopramide, 144
Middle ear. *See* Sinonasal passages/middle ear
Mints, 42, 72, 139, 144, 186
MTD (muscular tension dysphonia). *See also* Dysphonia
and globus sensation, 80-81
and LPR, 68, 73
Mucinex, 138
Mucus overproduction, 51, 52, 140, 167

N

Nasopharyngeal reflux (NPR)
diagnostic tests, 143-144
and FESS (functional endoscopic sinus surgery), 141-142
overview, 133-134, 137
NCCP (noncardiac chest pain). *See* Chest pain, noncardiac (NCCP)
NSAIDs (nonsteroidal anti-inflammatory drugs)
counterindicated, 144
and reflux, 139

O

Obesity, 51, 95, 136
Odynophagia, 4
Omeprazole
for asthma, 8
for chronic cough, 9-10
and chronic cough diagnosis, 109
for dysphagia, 152, 153, 156
for GERD/asthma outcomes, 99
for GERD with cough, 115, 120, 121-122
for laryngitis, 5, 111, 171
for LPR, 187, 189
for noncardiac chest pain, 11-12
for noncardiac chest pain (NCCP), 176
for sinonasal passages/middle ear involvement, 144
OSA (obstructive sleep apnea), 51
Otitis media (OM), 142-143
Otolaryngology: LPR, 49-60. *See also main heading* Laryngitis; *main heading* LPR (laryngopharyngeal reflux)
Over-the-counter (OTC) remedies, 56, 138-139
counterindicated, 144

P

Pantoprazole, 5, 42-43, 57, 171, 188
Pathophysiology
EERD
bile acids and pancreatic enzymes, 26
and differential diagnosis, 28
esophagotracheobronchial cough reflex, 26, 27
gastric acid and pepsin, 26
and laryngeal injury from GERD, 28-31
and LPR, 28-31
and lung injury from GERD, 26-28
nonacid reflux (NAR), 27-28, 31
overview, 26
tracheobronchial reflex, 26-27
GERD
acid and pepsin, 20
acid neutralization, esophageal clearance, 25
biliary and pancreatic secretions, 20-22

Pathophysiology: GERD *(continued)*
and EGF (epidermal growth factor), 25
epithelial defense/repair, 25
epithelial defense/repair, esophageal clearance, 25
esophageal clearance, 24-25
esophageal factors, 24-25
gastric emptying, 22
gastroduodenal factors, 20-22
gastroesophageal junction factors, 22-24
Helicobacter pylori, 22
hiatal hernia, 24
hypotensive LES, 23
nonacid reflux (NAR), 22
overview, 19-20, 25-26
pancreatic and biliary secretions, 20-22
pulmonary complaints, 26
TLESRs (transient LES relaxations), 22, 23
LPR, 38-39, 49-50, 56
pH
Bravo wireless pH monitoring system, 111
Pharyngeal reflux, 142
pH monitoring
and asthma, 7
Bravo wireless pH monitoring system, 125-127, 133, 143, 145, 178
esophageal, 111-113
globus sensation, 79-80
LPR (laryngopharyngeal reflux), 55-56
overview, 166
Restech Dx-pH Measurement System, 41
Physiology, sinonasal passages/middle ear, 135-137
Pitch anomalies, LPR, 68
Plausibility, biological
of asthma as EERD manifestation of GERD, 7
of chronic cough as EERD manifestation of GERD, 9
of laryngitis as EERD manifestation of GERD, 4-5
of noncardiac chest pain as EERD manifestation of GERD, 10-11
of tooth erosion as EERD manifestation of GERD, 12-13
Pneumonia, recurrent, 2
Polyps, laryngeal, 29
Postnasal drip (PND)
and chronic rhinosinusitis (CRS), 137-138
and cough, 108, 125, 173, 198
EERD (extraesophageal reflux disease), 134
and and globus sensation, 84
LPR, 38
Potassium, 139
PPIs. *See* Proton-pump inhibitors (PPIs)
Prevalence
of asthma as EERD manifestation of GERD, 6-7
of asthma (USA), 93
of chronic cough as EERD manifestation of GERD, 8-9, 26
of GERD, 1
GERD and asthma, 95
of laryngitis as EERD manifestation of GERD, 4
of noncardiac chest pain as EERD manifestation of GERD, 10
of tooth erosion as EERD manifestation of GERD, 95
of wheezing as EERD manifestation of GERD, 26
Prokinetic agents, 144
Proton-pump inhibitors (PPIs)
for asthma, 6-8, 97, 98, 101, 173
and cancer risk, 58-59
as chronic cough treatment, 9-10
combination/H2RA, 43-44, 113
and cough, chronic, 113
for dysphagia, 152, 153, 154-155, 156
and erosive esophagitis, 111
and esophageal clearance, 24-25
for esophageal spasm, 158
for GERD with cough, 114, 115, 116, 120, 121, 125, 127
and globus sensation, 85
for globus sensation, 87-88
for heartburn, 120
for laryngitis, 170, 171
as laryngitis treatment, 5-6
and LPR, 37, 39, 41-42, 42-44, 56-59

for LPR, 186–189
and NAB (nocturnal acid breakthrough), 44
for noncardiac chest pain (NCCP), 175–176
as noncardiac chest pain treatment, 11–12
PPI empiric trials, 168
for sinonasal passages/middle ear involvement, 144–145
and tooth erosion, 13
for tooth erosion, 13
Pseudoephephedrine, 138, 139–140
Pseudosulcus, laryngeal, 53, 69
Pulmonary diagnosis, 172
Pulmonary fibrosis, idiopathic, 2
Pulmonary symptoms, 6–10, 134
PVFM (paradoxical vocal fold movement), LPR, 68, 69–70, 73–74

Q

Quinidine, 139

R

Rabeprazole, 5, 11–12, 154–155, 171, 176, 187, 188
Ranitidine, 44, 120, 152, 153, 189
Regurgitation
and asthma, 94, 100
and EERD, 134
and eosinophilic esophagitis, 156
incidence of, 19
and LPR, 39
RFS (Reflux Finding Score)/LPR, 53–54, 58
Rhinosinusitis
acute bacterial, 138–139
chronic (CRS), 51
and FESS (functional endoscopic sinus surgery), 141–142
and gastric reflux, 141
histamine-2 receptor antagonists (H2RA), 144
overview, 137–138
postnasal drip (PND), 137–138
treatment, 139
overview, 137–140
symptoms/signs, 138
treatment, 138–139
RSI (Reflux Symptom Index)
actual form, 52
and globus sensation, 82
and LPR, 39, 40, 52, 58, 140–141

S

Scleroderma, 23, 157
Sedatives, 139
Sildenafil, 139
Sinonasal passages/middle ear
EERD, 133–145
diagnostic tests, 143–144
evidence supporting association, 140–143
otitis media (OM), 142–143
overview, 145
pharyngeal reflux, 142
treatment, 144–145
and *Helicobacter pylori,* 136–137
impedance matching, nasal airway/lungs, 135, 145
nasopharyngeal reflux (NPR), 133–134, 137, 141–142, 143–144
overview, 133–134
physiology, 135–137
postnasal drip (PND), 138
rhinosinusitis
acute bacterial, 138–139
chronic (CRS), 137–138 (*See also* chronic *under* Rhinosinusitis)
overview, 137–140
symptoms/signs, 138
treatment, 138–139
sinusitis, 136
Sinusitis
as EERD manifestation of GERD, 2
pathophysiology, 136
SLP role, LPR
breathing help, 73
cough help, 73–74
diet, 72
and lifestyle changes, 72
management, 68, 71
overview, 70, 72
treatments, 72–74
and vocal hygiene, 72

SLP role, LPR *(continued)*
vocal hyperfunction help, 73
voice rest/conservation, 72-73
voice therapy, 73
Smoking, 23, 25, 50–51, 68, 72, 110
Sore throat
as EERD manifestation of GERD, 2, 4
and LPR, 68
Speech-language pathology/pathologist. *See main heading* SLP role, LPR
Steroids, 138, 139, 140, 153
Subglottic stenosis
GERD, 107
LPR, 40, 51, 67
Sudafed, 139-140
Sulcus vocalis, 53
Surgery
and esophageal clearance, 24-25
FESS (functional endoscopic sinus surgery), 139, 141–142
fundoplication
asthma, 123
and dysphagia, 158–160
and EERD, 59
heartburn, 123
fundoplication, laparoscopic Nissen, 113
fundoplication, laparoscopic Nissen-Rossetti, 59
fundoplication, Nissen, 155, 158–160
fundoplication, Toupet, 158–160
for GERD/asthma outcomes, 100
GERD with cough, 116, 117–119, 122–125
for LPR disorders, 71
sinonasal passages/middle ear, 145
vagotomy, 110

T

Tachykinin NK-1 receptor antagonists, 97
Tetracycline, 138
Theophylline, 138, 140
Throat clearing
as EERD manifestation of GERD, 2, 4, 26
and LPR, 37, 38, 39, 51, 52, 68
Tooth erosion
biological plausibility, 12–13
and prevalence, 12, 95
treatment, 13
Transnasal endoscopy (TNE). *See also* Endoscopy
globus sensation, 87
LPR (laryngopharyngeal reflux), 55, 58
Transnasal laryngoscopy, LPR, 52–54
Treatment
acid suppression/EERD (extraesophageal reflux disease), 1, 6, 7–8, 9–10, 11–12, 13, 14
antimicrobial, 139
of asthma as EERD manifestation of GERD, 7–8, 14
asthma outcomes/GERD therapy, 98–100
breathing help, 73
of chronic cough as EERD manifestation of GERD, 9–10
chronic rhinosinusitis (CRS), 139
cough help, 73-74
diet, 72
dysphagia, 152, 154–155, 156, 158
GERD, 185-186
and cough, 114–127
globus sensation, 87–88
of laryngitis as EERD manifestation of GERD, 4–5
lifestyle changes, 72
LPR, 56–60, 186–190 (*See also main heading* LPR (laryngopharyngeal reflux))
dietary, 42, 56, 57
lifestyle modifications, 42, 56, 57, 72
PPIs, 42–44
LPR (laryngopharyngeal reflux), 37
respiratory retraining, 73
rhinosinusitis, 138–139
by SLPs
breathing help, 73
cough help, 73–74
diet, 72
lifestyle changes, 72
vocal hygiene, 72
vocal hyperfunction help, 73
voice rest/conservation, 72–73
voice therapy, 73
Triamcinolone, 153

U

URI (upper respiratory infection)
  and globus sensation, 85
  and laryngospasm, 60
  viral, 138

V

Valium, 139
VAPP (Voice Activity and Participation Profile), 72
VHI (Voice Handicap Index), 72
Viagra, 139
Videoendoscopy, esophagoglottal closure reflex, 30
Videostrobolaryngoscopy, 68-69
Vitamin supplements, 139
  counterindicated, 144

W

Wheezing, 26
  1q2wswbdexfcvgq

X

Xanthines, 138, 140